Influences in Health Care:
Media Perspectives

First edition February 1997

Published by
Macmillan Magazines Ltd
Porters South
4 Crinan Street
London N1 9XW

Companies and representatives throughout the world

Printed in Great Britain by
Grange Press
Southwick, West Sussex

ISBN 0 333 675355

CORE MEMBERS OF DEGREE TEAM

Cathy Hull, head of curriculum development and publishing, Macmillan Open Learning

Michelle Murtagh, editorial PA, Macmillan Open Learning

Elizabeth Redfern, education consultant (formerly assistant director for educational policy, English National Board)

Eimer Rogers, projects manager, Macmillan Open Learning

Simon Shaw, director, Cambridge Training and Development Ltd

DEGREE ADVISORY TEAM

Dai Hall, open and distance learning co-ordinator, Post Compulsory Education and Training, University of Greenwich

John Humphreys, head of school, Post Compulsory Education and Training, University of Greenwich

Debra Humphris, senior research fellow, Healthcare Evaluation Unit, St George's Hospital Medical School, London

Linda Husband, lecturer, Humberside College of Health and tutor/counsellor to Macmillan Open Learning DipHE students

Chris James, professor, University of Glamorgan Business School, formerly lecturer in education, Faculty of Education, University of Bath

Anne Palmer, education consultant to the University of Westminster

Richard Parish, chief executive and principal, Humberside College of Health

Marianne Phillips, head of division, Macmillan Open Learning, and University Pathway Director for DipHE

Frank Quinn, director of healthcare education, Post Compulsory Education and Training, University of Greenwich

Gwilym Roberts, director of fieldwork studies, School of Occupational Therapy, London Hospital Medical College, University of London

MACMILLAN OPEN LEARNING ADVISORY COMMITTEE

Margaret Alexander, professor, Department of Nursing and Community Health, Glasgow Caledonian University

Sue Frost, director of adult and children's nursing, English National Board

Liz Gillies, professional officer, National Board for Nursing, Midwifery and Health Visiting for Scotland

Maureen Lavery, professional officer, National Board for Nursing, Midwifery and Health Visiting for Northern Ireland

Ann Ryall-Davies, director of professional services, Welsh National Board for Nursing, Midwifery and Health Visiting

Jeff Thompson, CBE, professor, School of Education, University of Bath

INFLUENCES IN HEALTH CARE: MEDIA PERSPECTIVES — CONTRIBUTORS

Richard Hannaford, health correspondent, BBC London

David Miller, lecturer in film and media studies, Stirling University

Joanne Rule, director of external affairs, Royal College of Nursing, London

Jean Snedegar, freelance broadcaster and journalist

Jonathan Street, of Jonathan Street Public Relations Ltd, London

CRITICAL READERS FOR OVERALL DEGREE

Moya Davis, distance learning consultant and author

Anne Palmer, education consultant to the University of Westminster

Frank Quinn, director of healthcare education, Post Compulsory Education and Training, University of Greenwich

Gwilym Roberts, director of fieldwork studies, School of Occupational Therapy, London Hospital Medical College, University of London

CRITICAL READERS, INFLUENCES IN HEALTH CARE: MEDIA PERSPECTIVES UNIT

Mike Phillips, formerly senior lecturer in media studies, University of Westminster

Ian Wylie, head of communications, King's Fund, London

Di Marks-Maran, resource-based learning manager, Thames Valley University, London

Alan Howard, clinical nurse leader, psychosis (mental health), Bethlem Royal Hospital, Kent

STUDENT TESTERS

Audrey Gordon, student nurse, University of Abertay, Scotland

David Ingle, radiographer, London Chest Hospital

Claire Jackson, speech and language therapist, Kingston General Hospital, Hull

Ishbel Mackenzie, student nurse, University of Abertay, Scotland

EDITORIAL TEAM

Patsy Dale, chief sub-editor, Macmillan Open Learning

Cathy Hull, editor

Anne Rooney, writer

Simon Shaw, editor

DESIGN

Clare Conway, design studio, Macmillan Magazines

Graham Ogilvie, design studio, Macmillan Magazines

Steve Sullivan, graphic artist, Macmillan Magazines

Jane Walker, art director, Macmillan Magazines

PHOTOGRAPHS

Sue Lloyd, picture researcher, *Nursing Times*

Louise Thomas, picture researcher, *The Health Service Journal*

Special thanks to Medway NHS Trust for the use of their hospital as a photography resource

THE MACMILLAN OPEN LEARNING MISSION STATEMENT

The Macmillan Open Learning (MOL) programmes are based on the belief that the development of professional practice can be achieved only through the development of the professional as a person.

The MOL development team believe that:
- To become autonomous practitioners, professionals need to be self-directed, autonomous learners

- A programme of learning should focus on the learning process rather than the factual content

- The key to learning how to learn is through inquiry, reflection, evaluation and action

- An action-based, problem-solving approach to learning, combined with the reality of practice, will provide the appropriate stimulus and framework for learning.

Practice-based learning is the stimulus for raising standards of care generally within the learner's practice setting.

MOL programmes are therefore based on the following principles:
- A focus on learning rather than teaching

- Active involvement of learners, who have ownership of the learning, assessment and reflection processes

- Action-based, problem-solving approaches, which combine with the reality of practice to provide the stimulus and framework for learning

- Experiential approaches to learning which provide multiple and varied opportunities for learners to experience and/or act out the behaviours, knowledge and values of their own profession

- An emphasis on the integration of theory and practice in order that learners learn to structure concepts when thinking and making professional judgements in their practice.

Assessment is therefore integral to the learning process, rather than separate from it, and should:
- Enable and encourage learners to evaluate their own performance

- Focus on learners' critical analysis skills, and their ability to apply what has been learnt

- Enable and encourage learners to value personal theories and opinions.

CONTENTS

You and the book

This book contains the supporting material for one of the option units of the BSc (Hons) Professional Practice in Health Care. It gives an introduction to the role of the media in contemporary society and how their portrayal of healthcare issues affects the work of healthcare professionals.

The book presents theories about the function and influence of the media and gives examples of the ways in which the media report healthcare issues. It will help you find your way around the theories and learn to use them to understand the impact of the media. It also suggests opportunities to test them out through your own experience and practice.

If you are undertaking the degree programme, you will be doing two more option units as well as this one, and the core unit, *Enquiring Into Healthcare Practice*. The titles of the other option units are shown on the opposite page. You can study units separately, with support material in the form of a whole book (like this one) or as Professional Practice Study Units (PPSUs). Each PPSU contains one Section of a book. You can also buy a complete unit, with assessment, without having to register for a degree.

Studying PPSUs alone will enable you to develop some of the skills and capabilities you get from doing a degree. There are a number of advantages of studying several PPSUs:
- You will be able to study a topic in depth
- You will be able to appreciate the complexity of a topic from studying different approaches
- You will have the opportunity to synthesise knowledge from different sources
- By undertaking the assessment and the enquiry-based project you will have the opportunity to take the outcomes of a substantial, sustained piece of learning into practice.

For more information, contact:
Macmillan Open Learning
Porters South
Crinan Street
London N1 9XW

You probably had some good reasons for choosing to study this unit. You may want to write them down, or draw a picture or diagram of your initial impressions of the unit. If you do, your learning journal or reflective diary is a good place.

Your ideas may change as you work through the unit. Keep track of your thoughts and feelings by writing or drawing when you notice changes.

Testers of the material in this book said: 'When I looked at the book I wanted to do all the things in boxes first. Then I looked at the text in the upper half of the page. I read the top half with the questions and discussion points in mind, so when I looked at the boxes again, they seemed to mean more.'

'I've studied quite a bit by open learning. This programme seems to give me more freedom. I like the idea of not having to work through one Section completely before going on to the next, but instead being able to follow a train of thought.'

However you use the book, you are likely to find that it often doesn't provide answers but instead raises many questions. These may be just as important as answers. Take a few moments to think about the questions. If it is possible, talk about them with others at work or with your tutor/counsellor.

References are given in both the top and bottom halves of the pages. Follow up the references when you are investigating topics. Get to know the up-to-date, relevant literature as well.

One of the critical readers of this book said: 'The content and activities are highly topical and relevant. However students should be encouraged at the beginning to relate it to their own branch of health care and to make clear what their own intentions are in studying this unit. They need to think what the emphasis is going to be for their practice and learning.'

Taking charge

People learn in different ways, so use this book in a way that suits how you learn best. Some people like to start at the beginning and work through to the end. Others prefer a less systematic approach and like to take in different points of view as they go along. Links between Sections are built into the text, so you may find yourself going from one Section to another. There is no particular reason to read the various Sections in the order in which they are presented.

In general, it is more rewarding to decide for yourself how you will learn rather than have other people decide for you, and you can still achieve the assessment criteria if you are doing the degree (see pages 6-7).

Layout

The book has five Sections, with each Section divided into topics.

Most topics take up two facing pages – a double page spread. Read the book in this way – looking at both pages together as a whole. On many pages there is space for you to note your own views.

The top half of the page contains the kind of information which will stimulate you into researching and finding out more about the topic. The bottom half of the page has different sorts of information and gives you the opportunity to do something with it. There are activities, discussion points, quotes, references, charts, diagrams, current debates, case studies and ideas for assessment topics. However, you can read the bottom half of the page before the top half or mix them in any way that helps you to think and learn.

Boxes with dotted lines round them are Activity boxes, which contain material suggesting you do or think about some particular aspect relating to the text. Boxes that are tinted contain further references, quotes and comments.

Unit titles for the BSc(Hons) Professional Practice in Health Care

Core Unit: Enquiring into Healthcare Practice

Influences in Health Care: Media perspectives

Complementary Therapies and Healthcare Practice

Health Care and the Information Age

Health Promotion in Professional Practice

Healthcare Evaluation

Professional Relationships: Influences on health care

Values and the Person: Ideas that influence health care

As you work on this unit, draw your own links with topics that are covered in other units.

Learning and reflection

Reflective learning

When you are learning, it helps to reflect on the new ideas coming into your mind. You can do this by having a conversation with yourself, or with other people. But it is a particular sort of conversation: you will be asking questions, explaining, disagreeing, trying to get to the heart of the matter, turning things over in your mind, worrying about them. It could be useful to write some of this down, maybe in a learning journal or a reflective diary where you could be writing about:

- The process of learning
- The consequences of what has been learned
- What you discover about yourself as you learn.

Don't worry if things you read about in the book seem hazy for a time — that often happens when people are learning. Making notes and talking to others can help to clarify things and bring them into focus. Feed uncertainties into your writing and discussions, and into your personal profile as well (see pages 8-9).

Activities

When you come across an Activity, decide if you want to do it. You will be able to do some Activities if you are sitting on your own, reading, but not all of them. Many of the Activities give you something to go out and try in practice. You are more likely to do them if, for example:

- You are going to talk to other people about them — your tutor/counsellor or colleagues
- You are interested enough to have a conversation with yourself about them — what the Russian psychologist Vygotsky called 'internalised dialogue'
- You decide to save them up for later, when you have more time.

If you want to do an Activity, give yourself enough time and plan:

- When you are going to do it
- What else you will need, apart from time; for example, you might have to do some research or talk to a few people
- How you will keep a record of what you have done — this is so you can look at it later, or include it in your profile.

Reflection sometimes requires you to stand back from what you have been doing and make a deliberate effort to think about it. Talking or writing can help.

Think, talk or write about:

- What you just did, for example, tackled an Activity on your own, read a Section of the book, tried to talk to somebody
- Why you did it like that
- Where it seems to fit in with what you have done before
- What was good and bad about it
- How you felt about it
- What it made you think.

What are the consequences?

- Describe the situation
- Ask yourself why it happened the way it did
- Think about how it was different from what you expected
- Work out what to do next.

You may want to keep track of what you have read in the book. Devise a system of marking the book to help you. There is a box next to each heading on the contents page which you could tick when you have read the topic. Or you could highlight the boxes to show which topics you want to investigate in more depth.

Apollinaire said

'Come to the edge'

'But it is too high'

'Come to the edge'

'We might fall'

'Come to the edge'

And they came

And he pushed them

And they flew

4

You might decide to keep an Activity log as a record of your intentions and what you achieved by doing the Activities.

Integrating learning into practice

As you study this unit, or the degree programme as a whole, you will be learning general things as well as specific knowledge related to the unit topics. Your learning should integrate into practice. Many descriptions of the professional role emphasise the importance of continual learning. One study looking at the links between degree-level education and practice (Winter, 1994) identified that the professional role includes these four things:

- A requirement that understanding should continually develop through reflection upon practice
- Interpretative responsibility towards an always incomplete body of knowledge
- A basis in a complex set of ethical principles
- An understanding of the importance of affective dimensions (conscious and unconscious)

Another study looking at evidence of capability in a professional context (Eraut, 1994) found that the professional role includes:

- Understanding clients
- Analysing problems and situations
- Discussing the relative merits of alternative approaches
- Evaluating the professional practice you observe
- Conceptualising and evaluating your own work in order to learn from experience
- Creating knowledge.

The study also emphasised the value of having underlying knowledge of techniques (including those still at pilot stage) and a critical understanding of:

- The concepts, theories and principles which underpin current practice
- The significance of innovations
- The role played by your profession in society.

What does being a professional mean to you?

You might like to compare your thoughts with those expressed in the literature issued by your relevant statutory, professional or self-regulating body.

'When a practitioner becomes a researcher into his own practice, he engages in a continuing process of self-education.' Schön, D. (1991) *The Reflective Practitioner: How professionals think in action.* Aldershot, Hants: Avebury Press:

'"I didn't realise I knew so much. I didn't realise I could do so much". This is the sort of statement often made by people who have spent some time evaluating their jobs.' Hull, C. (1992) Making experience count: facilitating the APEL process. In: Griffin, C. and Mulligan, J. (eds) *Empowerment through Experiential Learning.* London: Kogan Page.

Do you have an appropriate sense of what you do and what you know?

Use a journal or reflective diary as a way of evaluating what you do and what you need to know in order to do it.

Assessment guidelines

This unit can be used to gain credits towards a BSc degree programme. To gain credit you will need to do some work that can be assessed. It is a good idea to start thinking about assessment right now. *You* can take charge of assessment — within the limits of the BSc programme and what you agree with your tutor/counsellor after negotiation.

If you wish to undertake the degree you will need to show that you can:
- Critically reflect on and challenge existing practice
- Draw on perspectives from within and beyond your own professional boundaries and use these to inform your own practice, where appropriate
- Develop and extend your own professional knowledge and skills through a process of analysis, synthesis and evaluation of the contemporary theoretical concepts that underpin current practice
- Plan, conduct and evaluate an enquiry-based project related to your field of practice
- Critically reflect on and evaluate your own personal, professional development and learning.

These are the overall learning outcomes for the degree as a whole. You should demonstrate that you have achieved them all throughout your work on the degree, including the unit assessments and the enquiry-based project.

The specific learning outcomes for this unit require you to:
- Discuss the origins and development of media interest in health care from a number of perspectives
- Critically review the role of the media in influencing health care and professional practice
- Evaluate your own personal and professional practice in relation to understanding and influencing the media.

To gain credits towards the degree, you will need to produce a written assessment which shows that you have achieved all the learning outcomes. In the assessment you will critically analyse the role and impact of the media on a number of aspects of your professional practice. It is up to you to decide what you want to write about. Negotiate with your tutor/counsellor the exact wording of your assessment title.

There is a game about assessment with five stages. Playing the game shows what it is like when you can negotiate the assessment process. It is played in a group of 12 or more.

Stage 1 – One person is asked to stand up and clap, then leave the room.

Stage 2 – Four or five people are given a clapping score sheet and asked to act as an assessment panel. They have to decide individual criteria for assessing how well people clap. Next, another person is asked to stand up and clap, and then leaves the room. Each member of the panel awards the clapper a score out of five.

Stage 3 – Members of the panel get together to agree their criteria for assessing how well people clap. The next person is asked to stand up and clap and leaves the room while the panel agrees what score to award. The clapper is told the score but is not told what it means.

Stage 4 – The next person is told the criteria before being asked to clap. That person is also told the final score, together with an explanation.

Stage 5 – The last clapper is asked to sit down and have a chat about clapping. The panel acknowledges that the clapper has some knowledge of the subject and they ask what criteria the clapper would like to be assessed against. The criteria are agreed and the person is asked to clap when ready. The clapper is asked for an opinion of the performance. After a brief discussion, the panel then describes how they would assess the performance and a final score is negotiated by the panel and the clapper.

How do you think each of the clappers in the game described above might feel?

Which one would you rather be?

What do you think the game shows about different ways of assessing performance?

If you have registered for the degree, you will also be working on an enquiry-based project. This is a major piece of research including a written assessment. The core unit for the BSc degree, entitled *Enquiring into Healthcare Practice*, gives you guidance on how to carry out the project. Your work on other units, as well as this one on media, may give you ideas for topics to cover in the enquiry-based project. Talk to your tutor/counsellor about any practical details to do with assessment and refer for guidance to the university's regulations which accompany these materials.

Developing an assessment topic

At first, you may not have a clear idea of what you want to write about in your assessment. However, you should start developing your ideas early on as you learn about the role and impact of the media. When you feel that you have got the germ of an idea, start talking about it with other people — healthcare professionals, friends, your tutor/counsellor. If you don't feel ready to talk to other people, have a conversation — or several conversations — with yourself. Or write things down in your learning journal or reflective diary.

Don't worry if your ideas change a lot. But, sooner or later, you should put them down on paper and start to define the subject and scope of your assessment. Then negotiate the exact wording of the assessment with your tutor/counsellor.

The assessment habit

Get into the habit of continually assessing your work on this unit. Assessing yourself isn't only about deciding a topic for and completing the written assessment. People assess themselves all the time, often without realising it. They assess their behaviour, their moods, the way other people see them, the way they do things . . . One of the purposes of assessment is to help you learn, to clarify your reasons for learning certain things and to gauge how far you are getting. It can give you:

- Motivation — a reason for learning
- Practice — the opportunity to try things out
- Feedback — other people's comments on how you are doing
- Opportunity for reflection — time to think about what you have learned and how you have learned it, so as to build new knowledge into your existing practice.

Educational assessment is one of many forms of assessment which go on all the time. When you bake a cake you assess its success — how it looks, how it tastes, whether people like it. When you have a conversation you assess how the other person is responding to what you say. Derek Rowntree identifies the following, more formal kinds of assessment in addition to everyday conversational dialogue:

- Medical diagnosis
- The writing of biography
- Forensic cross-questioning
- Job interviews and promotion appraisals
- Criticism of the arts
- Refereeing of books and papers submitted for publication by scholarly journals.

'Such forms of assessment will sometimes offer revealing parallels and contrasts with those common in education.' Rowntree, D. (1977) *Assessing Students: How shall we know them?* London: Kogan Page.

You can negotiate an assessment topic with your tutor/counsellor. It is important that the topic allows you to demonstrate your understanding of the theory underpinning your work and to meet the learning outcomes.

As well as the written assessment, you might like to submit additional evidence, perhaps in one of the following forms:

- A video or tape recording plus a written critique of what is in it and how it was made

- A series of photographs or drawings with a similar written explanation

- An action plan or a design for evaluating an aspect of practice

- A set of comparative data, including statistics and other forms of numerical presentation.

The personal profile

Assessment in the wider sense helps to keep track of your personal and professional development during your studies. One way of capturing parts of this process is to keep a personal profile. The profile can provide you with a rich source of reflective material to be drawn on when planning and producing the written assessment. Use the profile to record your thoughts about how learning and assessment fit together.

The profile can draw on all your experiences and encompass many different kinds of writing. If you are keeping a learning journal, reflective diary or activity log, they can form part of the profile. This kind of informal writing will help you to articulate what Donald Schön calls 'knowing in action' (Schön, D., 1987). It also gives you the chance to use your imagination to look at different possibilities without having to risk trying things out in reality.

Writing, reflection and learning feed into one another. As you examine your work, writing your thoughts down will help you to make connections between learning, feeling and doing. This kind of informal writing helps you discover what you think about complex topics and will help you write better formal assessments.

What is profiling?

Profiling helps you (and others) make sense of what you are learning and relate it to your professional and personal life. It is a structured approach for reflecting on:

- Yourself
- Your abilities
- Different aspects of your life and work — including your career and professional development to date
- Plans for the future.

It will help you:

- Understand the complexity of your work
- Analyse your experience and view it more critically
- Appreciate your own professional development
- Value the extent of your learning.

Profiling means keeping a record of these things, organised in a way that is clear to you. Most profiles involve quite a lot of writing, because this is a good way of keeping a record and because writing things down often helps you clarify them in your mind. Writing can also help you make connections between different aspects of your life and learning.

There are many different materials which make up a profile, for example:

- A learning journal
- A reflective diary
- An activity log
- A reading log
- An action planner . . .

It doesn't matter what you call these materials as long as you write regularly and keep track of your thoughts and ideas.

Reflection involves 'creating stops in which one stands aside from one's own process and has a look to see what is happening.' Brazier, D. (1995) *Zen Therapy*. London: Constable.

Find time every so often to let your thoughts catch up with you. Give them a bit of space inside your head and let them speak to you. One of the good things about learning is that, given the chance, you will discover new thoughts that have formed themselves without your even knowing it.

What do you understand by the term 'critically review'? Draw on perspectives from outside your own professional boundaries when you are thinking about this question.

What do you understand by terms such as 'origins and development of media interest in health care'?

Where can you go to share ideas about questions such as these?

'I shall be telling this with a sigh,

Somewhere ages and ages hence:

Two roads diverged in a wood, and I –

I took the one less travelled by,

And that has made all the difference.'

Frost, R. (1951) 'The Road Not Taken.' *The Complete Poems of Robert Frost*, London: Jonathan Cape.

You will find suggestions on how to write things down, and where, as you work through this book; for example, in learning journals, reflective diaries, activity logs.

Other ways of keeping a record and thinking things through include drawing, taking photographs and recording on cassette significant conversations with other people. These can all form part of a profile and can be a good alternative to different forms of writing.

Whose profile is it?

Your personal profile is mainly for you. It will be a unique record of you as a learner. This means that you have control over where to start and what to include. There are no right or wrong ways. Some people prefer to start by keeping a reflective diary. Others start with a record of their professional education and training. Before you work on your profile you might find it useful to discuss it with a colleague, friend or tutor/counsellor. Identifying the different ways of using your profile will help you decide where and how you would like to start.

You may want to show some of it to other people as well. For example, if you have been thinking through a particular aspect of health-care evaluation that links closely to your work or your assessment, you may want to photocopy your notes, diagrams and ideas and discuss them with your tutor/counsellor or colleagues.

Macmillan Open Learning publishes a profile pack and workbook giving guidance on how to keep and use a profile. The handbook called *A Student's Guide to Open Learning* also contains a section on profiling. Both are available from Macmillan Open Learning at the address listed on page 2.

Profiling will help you as an individual to:
- Understand and appreciate the significance of what and how you learn
- Enhance your self-awareness and build confidence in the value of your experiences.

Profiling will help you as a professional to:
- Keep an effective and up-to-date record of your past and current learning
- Provide you with a powerful means of communication with your employers, present and future.

Think about keeping track of your reading in a learning journal. Whenever you read a book, a newspaper or journal article, write down your response to what you have read, any ideas which caught your imagination, questions that arose, further reading to be done. Your reading does not need to be confined to your subject area. Follow your interests and read widely. Parts of your journal might give you ideas for your written assessment.

Here are some guidelines for keeping track of reading:

- Read and write with some purpose in mind. Say why you selected a book or an article and what, overall, you learned from it, before taking issue with particular content.

- Focus on things which strike you or are intriguing to you in some way

Nightingale, P. (1986) *Improving Student Writing*. Kensington, New South Wales: Higher Education Research and Development Society of Australasia.

There could be two types of material in your profile:

- Confidential — that which is for your eyes only

- Professional — information about your learning and professional development that you are happy to share with others.

If you have started a profile for other purposes, you can continue using it for this unit.

Learning contracts

A learning contract is the sort of contract you can continually revise. It is not a binding legal document. The idea of a contract is to set out an agreement between two or more people — in this case, you and your tutor/counsellor. One of the things about a contract is that it helps you clarify your ideas, select realistic objectives and keep track of changes. Contracts don't have to be written down, although they usually are because writing down what you are intending to do is likely to help you develop planning and writing skills.

The work you do in your personal profile should lead you towards making a learning contract. As you think about what you have done in the past and what you are doing now, your thoughts will move to the future. Most people have both short-term and long-term goals. The profile is a good place to make notes of your plans and goals. Make these as specific as possible. You can refine them as you try new approaches and techniques. When you are happy, transfer them to the learning contract. If you use action plans as well, you have a very good system for monitoring your progress. If you find yourself straying too far from your goals, make some adjustments, both to your course and to your contract.

There is no one right way to construct a learning contract. People learn and speak and write in different ways. You might have to try out several approaches before finding the one that suits you best. On the page opposite you will see two different approaches.

'It is important to remember that no one has the right to read your portfolio without your permission. The UKCC reminds registrants that "your portfolio contains confidential information about you and should, therefore, not be accessible to others without your permission".

'When deciding whether to give your permission, you need to understand the person's reasons for wanting to read your portfolio. Knowing the reason behind their request will enable you to select parts of your portfolio that are relevant to their interest.'

Hull, C. and Redfern, E. (1996) *Profiles and Portfolios. A guide for nurses and midwives.* Basingstoke: Macmillan.

A lifeline (or road of life) is a picture of your professional and/or personal life. It shows both highs and lows as well as important events. It can contain a little or a lot of information.

Draw a road of life showing how you came to be doing this unit or the degree programme.

- How are events related?

- Where are the turning points?

As you go through the programme, think about how it is affecting your professional and personal life.

- What causes the highs?

- At what points do the lows occur?

Keep drawing the line as you go through the programme, and afterwards.

LEARNING CONTRACT

Re: Section 2
What do I need to do?
1 Use the next three weeks to work through the unit.
2 Plan time in my diary to visit the library to follow up references.
3 Attend group tutorial.
4 Make one appointment with tutor/counsellor to discuss ideas I have about my assessment.

What am I trying to learn from this Section?
(to be discussed with tutor/counsellor after group tutorial)

1 Need to look more closely at the question of media bias. Spoke to Cathy who used to work for the BBC World Service. She said that the BBC tries to maintain a balance in its reporting. I will do a literature search for articles about bias and objectivity.

2 During Section 1, I found myself skipping some of the suggested Activities. It didn't seem to matter at first, but Jenny seems to get much more out of the material by doing them. I'll set myself a target to do 50% of them for Section 2.

LEARNING CONTRACT

This is the first time I've ever learnt this way and I keep getting lost and feeling I'm not achieving anything. A colleague suggested I make a definite plan – what I'm going to learn and then agree it with my tutor/counsellor. I decided to try it for Sections 1 and 2.

1 Go through, page by page, and mark up any references I need to follow up.
   Action: Book time to go to the library
2 Use the models of mass communication as a framework for critical reflection on the media.
   Action: Have a look at McQuail's book.
3 See if I can find out where reporters get their information for a healthcare story, like the one on drug abuse in last week's papers. I wonder if they get it from articles in professional journals or direct from researchers?
   Action: Analyse drug abuse stories and compare to articles in professional journals.
4 Want to talk to a healthcare journalist. See if my tutor/counsellor can arrange this for me.
   Action: Prepare a list of questions to ask in advance.
5 Need to learn about how really to read and evaluate articles I find. It's difficult to know whether they are right or wrong.
   Action: Need to think about how I can do that.

Remember these general principles for evidence of your learning:

- Relevance — your learning must be relevant to the subject you are aiming to study or the award you are seeking
- Breadth — the learning you are demonstrating should relate to a wide body of knowledge and skills, particularly in the context of your own professional practice
- Currency — the learning you are showing must be up to date and relevant to your current working practices
- Authenticity — the evidence you provide must be your own work.

When assessing your life and learning, the following elements are involved:

- Your learning and your experience
- Reflecting upon your past learning
- Identifying significant learning
- Providing evidence of learning
- Direct evidence — things you produce yourself
- Indirect evidence — things other people say on your behalf.

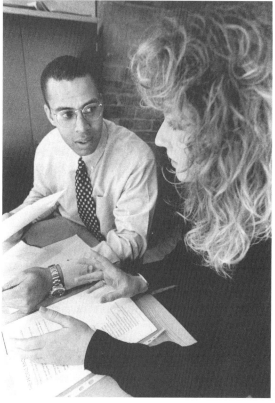

RICHARD SMITH

Perspectives on the media

The media consist of 'channels (for example, newspapers, radio, television) through which information is transmitted to the public' (*Chambers Dictionary*, 1993). On-line media such as the Internet and World Wide Web are also included. In today's culture, the media are a constant source of information, comment, opinion and entertainment. It is virtually impossible for anyone to ignore them or to avoid being influenced in some way by the messages they convey.

Strategies for coping with the media

People have developed mental strategies for dealing with this constant input. Some of the strategies have seeped into everyday language: people 'tune in' to things they want to hear, or 'switch off' when they are not paying attention. We have become sophisticated interpreters of messages, able to switch our attention rapidly from one subject to another and to differentiate between the many different kinds of messages we receive. We are able to take perspectives on the media, just as they adopt different perspectives on the events they report and mediate.

In some mediaeval paintings, many events are depicted together so that the painting has no single focus or perspective: there is no single way of looking at the events they record. For the mediaeval painter and viewer, this portrayed the rich diversity of experience and showed how the meaning of one event depends on knowledge and understanding of other, related events. To understand contemporary media requires a similar approach. It may seem as though individual stories or programmes follow a narrative and linear model: there is often a train of events, which follows a chronological sequence. But this linearity is more apparent than real. In fact, the way our minds absorb media messages is more like the way you might build up a mosaic, piece by piece, until the picture is complete.

Health care and the media

Health and illness are favourite media themes. They appear in countless news items, documentaries, soap operas and drama. Images of hospitals, doctors, midwives, other healthcare professionals and patients are constantly flickering on and off television screens. This increased exposure challenges healthcare professionals in a number of ways. For instance,

'People react to the media differently from the way they react to events in real life. Why do they find different things acceptable? For example, I regularly have students passing out on viewing a film on would healing, but none of them passed out on viewing a real wound. Do the media have additional effects, such as making things appear more gory than they really are? I can view the most horrendous injuries in real life or on film but can't watch *Doctor Who* without having nightmares. Where does that leave our neat and tidy idea that the media represent reality?'

Nurse educator

People develop an active, often critical relationship with the media. The people who wrote this book have ways of getting on with the media which influenced what they wrote. You have your own relationship and it is sure to be different. So don't take for granted anything you read here. Quarrel with it, disagree, look at the way you handle the media, scrutinise your own response.

The boxes below outline the contents of each Section of this book

Section 1 - Health Care and the Media

Introduces what the media are, what — and who — they report and the different perspectives they take when reporting events and issues related to health care. The Section also introduces some of the critical reading and analysis techniques needed to understand how the media operate.

Section 2 - Understanding the Media

Looks at how the media work on a day-to-day basis — researching and writing articles, producing programmes, designing publications. The Section also investigates influences, controls and regulations on the media. Several theoretical models of how the media work within society to influence and reflect opinion are introduced.

patients/clients may have expectations of the service that cannot be matched in reality; images of how doctors, nurses and other healthcare practitioners behave may not be accurate or appropriate; healthcare professionals may find themselves in the media front line. Understanding how the media work will help prepare healthcare professionals for working in a health service which is in the spotlight.

In this book you will find several topics and case studies for analysis. They have been chosen because they have received extensive media coverage and there is a lot to learn from how the media treated them. By looking closely at the way the media handled these cases you will build up a many-faceted picture of how healthcare issues are reported and the influences of these reports. You will also be asked to collect your own examples of media stories and events which you can analyse using the tools you develop as you work on the book. This will enable you more easily to demonstrate the ways in which you have made sense of the media and developed critical tools for analysing what you see, read and hear.

References

Eraut, M. (1994) Implications for standards development. In: *Competence and Assessment Compendium No.3*. London: Department of Employment.

Schön, D. (1987) *Educating the Reflective Practitioner*. San Francisco: Jossey-Bass.

Winter, R. (1994) The ASSET Programme - Competence-based education at professional/honours degree level. In: *Competence and Assessment Compendium No.3*. London: Department of Employment.

Key texts for this unit

Berger, J. (1990) *Ways of Seeing*. Harmondsworth: Penguin Books.

Bridges, J.M. (1990) Literature review on the images of the nurse and nursing in the media. London: *Journal of Advanced Nursing* 15 (7): 850–854.

Curran, J., Seaton, J. (1992) *Power Without Responsibility*. London: Routledge.

Hartley, J. (1992) *Understanding News*. London: Methuen. (Reprinted 1988, Routledge, London.)

Karpf, A. (1988) *Doctoring the Media – The reporting of health and medicine*. London: Routledge.

Philo, G. (1994) The impact of mass media on public images of mental illness: media content and audience belief. *Health Education Journal* 53 (3): 271–281.

Platt, S. (1987) The aftermath of Angie's overdose: Is soap (opera) damaging to your health. *British Medical Journal* 294: 954–957.

Section 3 - Influences on the Media

Focuses on the interplay of public demand and the constraints of production on the media. The first part of the Section looks at the different forms of printed and broadcast media which are likely to carry healthcare coverage. The second part looks at the ways in which health care is represented and the types of topic that come up in different media forms.

Section 4 - The Impact on Healthcare Practice

Looks at how people respond to coverage of health care in the media, ranging from the careful attention given to a professional journal to the far more casual engagement with a television programme watched by chance. This Section also examines the social impact of the media and its effect on policy.

Section 5 - Getting Across the Message

Shows how to make the shift from looking at the media from the outside to taking the perspective of an insider. The Section also provides practical techniques for healthcare professionals to engage successfully with the media, by making the most of interviews, press conferences and press releases.

Introduction

The media are the means by which communication is made to huge numbers of people at the same time — mass communication. Newspapers, radio, television, films, videos, magazines, journals, the Internet are all examples of media. The media penetrate people's lives with images and representations covering the spectrum of human experience, so it is not surprising that health care features extensively: it is covered in news stories about epidemics, scandals and scares, medical developments or nurses' pay. It is also the subject of documentaries on medical procedures and illnesses, live broadcasts from hospitals, dramas and films staged in healthcare settings. Characters in soap operas respond to and worry about illness, while newspaper and magazine articles about environmental conditions or political and economic policy often reflect on the implications for health.

What impact does the exposure of health issues have on the public and on healthcare professionals? It means that patients and clients develop their own ideas of what to expect from the health service and can therefore make criticisms of how treatment could be handled. Furthermore, it means they may cast themselves in different roles; for example as victims in the hands of doctors, consumers of healthcare services, or campaigners against cutbacks and poor service.

Why it matters

We live with the media and our attitudes, values and beliefs are intertwined with the things we read, see and hear. But do the media really matter? In what ways do they shape and influence our lives — and do they change things or simply reflect the changes made by others? As you work on this book you will be thinking about:

- Who influences the media
- How accurate and objective it is
- How stories are picked up by the media and shaped by different influences
- How the health service uses and responds to the media
- How the media may impact on health care directly.

You will be analysing your own response to the way health is covered in the media and thinking about how this may affect people's views and expectations. You will also be exploring the complex ways in which people relate to the media and interact with them.

One way of reading newspapers and magazines, listening to the radio or watching television is as a leisure pursuit. It tends to be 'down time' for the brain. But to get the most out of this book, you should not be passive. Be an active reader, viewer and listener and an informed critic of the media. Do not let messages seep in and influence you without analysing and judging them. Challenge every broadcast and every press article by asking questions such as:

- Whose views are portrayed?
- Why are they given space or air time?
- How will the piece appear to an uninitiated viewer or reader, and how will it appear to one who shares the knowledge on which it is based?
- What is the message the writer or broadcaster wants to communicate?
- Is the intended message the one you receive and do you accept and agree with it?

'Arguably the power of the media has increased remarkably in the last forty years. There are fewer alternative sources of information, while the control of the media has become concentrated in fewer hands. At the same time the press and broadcasting have become less accountable. The public means of monitoring performance is wholly incapable of coping with growth and technological change in increasingly complex industries.'

Curran, J. and Seaton, J. (1991) *Power Without Responsibility. The press and broadcasting in Britain* (4th edition). London: Routledge.

What's in the media?

News and features

People generally expect the news to be presented without the intervention of anyone's point of view — the 'facts'. But raw facts are meaningless. They must be put into some context, subjected to some form of selection and presented in a shape that gives them meaning. Some writers and broadcasters try hard to produce material with as little bias as possible. But because language is never neutral or transparent, there is necessarily some interpretation going on even in the most unbiased news report. As you work through this book you will be learning how to distinguish between facts and their interpretation and presentation.

Controversial subjects are often presented as irreconcilable. This is partly because the media give a roughly equal amount of time to the arguments and partly because issues are reduced to the level of personalities — politicians in particular are often presented in a series of short soundbites (see pages 108–111 for more on how the media present politicians). Over time, this type of presentation can become a ritual balancing act which alienates people who are not closely involved with the issues.

To read between the lines of the ritual, people need to develop their own internal mechanisms for understanding the codes. For example, a politician who says on the TV news that 'the welfare state should be used by people who need it' may be giving a coded message that the social service budget is about to be cut because some people are benefiting who do not need help. Nowhere in the bulletin is there any exploration of what is meant by the word 'need'. Viewers have two choices: they can switch off or they can engage their critical faculties to crack the code and scrutinise what is really being said.

Features

In a documentary or feature, whether in a broadcast or print medium, there has been more time to collect and collate information, check sources and find other relevant material for comparison and support. Documentaries and features have a 'line' — a point other than just reporting what has happened. They aim to interpret events and find meaning in what may have been covered in the news but has since been assimilated and analysed. We expect comment and interpretation as well as facts; there may be no topical content at all.

'Fiction is a form of discourse, which, under guise of invention, illustrates or proves an idea; and, as its superficial aspect is removed, the meaning of the author is clear.'

Boccaccio, G. *Genealogia deorum gentilium*, Book 14, Sections ix and x, translated by Osgood, C.G. (1930) *Boccaccio on Poetry*. Princeton: Princeton University Press.

'What is an alternative to the way arguments are presented on the media? Rather than looking for differences — black and white — we could start by looking for the common ground. After that we can focus on the points where arguments diverge. Actually, that gets closer to what happens in politics and to the decision-making process. Quite often politicians start with a lot of common ground.'

Councillor Vernon Hull, leader, Medway City Council.

You might like to look up some of the important words you come across as you work on this book and other parts of your course. You could begin with 'media' and 'communications'. A useful source of information on how meanings accrue and change as a word is used in the language is:

Williams, R. (1983). *Keywords*. London: Fontana (second edition).

How true to life does fiction have to be? Think of a novel or TV fiction you have read or watched recently. How did you 'remove its superficial aspect'? What did you discover underneath? You might like to make notes in your reflective diary as you go along.

Fiction

People often expect fiction to be true to life. Expectations of fiction are linked to genre. For example, in a science fiction film, it is normal to accept implausible technology as this is one of the conventions (and one of the appeals) of the form. But audiences generally expect realism in the responses of the human characters to the unfamiliar situations in which they find themselves. If the characters are implausible audiences may lose confidence and interest in the film.

For a hospital drama to be credible it needs to give a realistic portrayal of the events that occur within a hospital, show realistic relationships between staff and between staff and patients, and give accurate representations of medical conditions. Viewers may accept improbability within certain bounds (such as a large number of interesting incidents in a single day) but not in those areas which engage their sympathy and interest — these must remain realistic or people cannot easily identify with them. The bounds may be quite wide — for example, what relevance might there be to healthcare professionals in a piece of fiction such as Mary Shelley's *Frankenstein* (or its film version)?

Audrey: 'I do not know what "poetical" is. Is it honest in deed and word? Is it a true thing?'

Touchstone: 'No, truly; for the truest poetry is the most feigning...'

Shakespeare, *As You Like It*. Act 3, Scene 3.

How well do fictional TV programmes reflect your profession?

Bringing it together

As you work on the Activities in this book you will be taking pieces from the media out of context: an article snipped out of a paper or magazine, or text from a video- or audiotape or a broadcast. Doing this, there is a danger of losing sight of the context in which the material was originally presented. You may need to remind yourself of the context. This is important because the components of a publication or set of programmes make up a complex construct in which each item has its own meaning and the interrelations between items also have meaning. The media are more than the sum of their parts. An article or programme gets extra dimensions of meaning from its conjunction with surrounding material, including advertising, the layout or presentation style and the overall flavour or tone of its context. So the pieces you are studying in isolation would normally have been received and interpreted in the context of the surrounding matter.

For a week keep a note of all forms of the broadcast and print media you look at. Record:

- What you looked at, for example, *The Independent*.
- The type of material you looked at — news coverage, features, fiction, advertisements
- How long you spent looking at it, for example half an hour watching a comedy on TV, 15 minutes flicking through a magazine
- The situation in which you looked at it — listening to the radio while making breakfast, reading the paper on the train
- How much you remembered later of what you saw, heard or read.

See if a pattern emerges over the week. Which media do you use most? To which do you give your full attention? What type of material are you most likely to receive passively and which actively? What makes the difference?

Perspectives in media images

When you watch a broadcast or look at a photograph in a newspaper or magazine, it is revealing to think about the point of view or perspective it is promoting. Camera angle, lighting, the background, the positions of the people and all elements of the picture's composition contribute to its meaning and effect. Its relationship to other images or text can also add to or alter the meaning the picture would have if looked at in isolation.

Reading images

In the adjacent column are two photographs of a politician. One shows her in a casual pose and clothes, the other in formal dress. In one she is with her family, in the other she is with other politicians. It would not be necessary to read the accompanying news report to guess the type of article each picture illustrates. The first says 'family matters' or 'positive PR job'; the second supports a story about official business.

Body language and dress codes are both ways of creating an image. Politicians use them skilfully — they are trained to know what they will look like when a camera is pointed at them. Media pictures often use a sort of iconographic shorthand. Particular images call up resonances

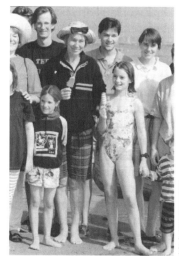

Unofficial business

SOLO SYNDICATION

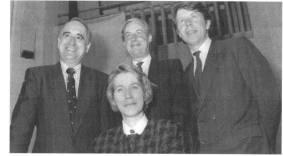

Official business

PHILIP WOLMUTH

THE GUARDIAN

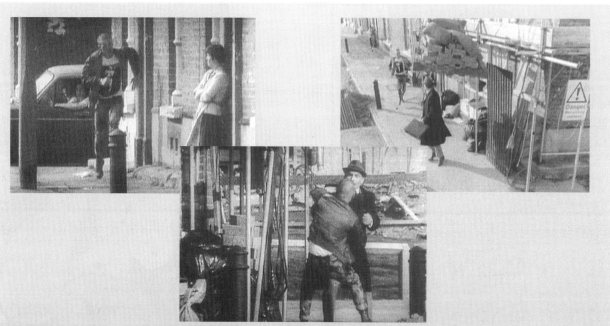

What is included in a picture helps to define its meaning. This series of images is from a television advertisement for the *Guardian*. The scene in the centre looks like a mugging — the dress and appearance of the man endorse this reading. We may make assumptions about people based on factors like these. In fact the man in the bomber jacket is saving the old man from a potential accident (centre picture). The sequence makes us analyse our assumptions about people as well as think about how selectivity can change the meaning of a picture.

Fiction

People often expect fiction to be true to life. Expectations of fiction are linked to genre. For example, in a science fiction film, it is normal to accept implausible technology as this is one of the conventions (and one of the appeals) of the form. But audiences generally expect realism in the responses of the human characters to the unfamiliar situations in which they find themselves. If the characters are implausible audiences may lose confidence and interest in the film.

For a hospital drama to be credible it needs to give a realistic portrayal of the events that occur within a hospital, show realistic relationships between staff and between staff and patients, and give accurate representations of medical conditions. Viewers may accept improbability within certain bounds (such as a large number of interesting incidents in a single day) but not in those areas which engage their sympathy and interest — these must remain realistic or people cannot easily identify with them. The bounds may be quite wide — for example, what relevance might there be to healthcare professionals in a piece of fiction such as Mary Shelley's *Frankenstein* (or its film version)?

Audrey: 'I do not know what "poetical" is. Is it honest in deed and word? Is it a true thing?'

Touchstone: 'No, truly; for the truest poetry is the most feigning...'

Shakespeare, *As You Like It*. Act 3, Scene 3.

How well do fictional TV programmes reflect your profession?

Bringing it together

As you work on the Activities in this book you will be taking pieces from the media out of context: an article snipped out of a paper or magazine, or text from a video- or audiotape or a broadcast. Doing this, there is a danger of losing sight of the context in which the material was originally presented. You may need to remind yourself of the context. This is important because the components of a publication or set of programmes make up a complex construct in which each item has its own meaning and the interrelations between items also have meaning. The media are more than the sum of their parts. An article or programme gets extra dimensions of meaning from its conjunction with surrounding material, including advertising, the layout or presentation style and the overall flavour or tone of its context. So the pieces you are studying in isolation would normally have been received and interpreted in the context of the surrounding matter.

For a week keep a note of all forms of the broadcast and print media you look at. Record:

- What you looked at, for example, *The Independent*.
- The type of material you looked at — news coverage, features, fiction, advertisements
- How long you spent looking at it, for example half an hour watching a comedy on TV, 15 minutes flicking through a magazine
- The situation in which you looked at it — listening to the radio while making breakfast, reading the paper on the train
- How much you remembered later of what you saw, heard or read.

See if a pattern emerges over the week. Which media do you use most? To which do you give your full attention? What type of material are you most likely to receive passively and which actively? What makes the difference?

Fact and fiction

Much of the portrayal of healthcare settings and professionals on television is fiction — drama, film, situation comedy and serials. The billing a programme is given indicates whether viewers should interpret it as fact or fiction: *Panorama* is expected to deal in true facts, *Casualty* is expected to show realistic, though not historically real, happenings. But it may be harder than it looks for people to separate fact from fiction in what they see on television. The judgement they make will depend partly on how alert they are at the time and partly on how well informed they are about the issues. A nurse who has worked in an accident and emergency department might say that *Casualty* is unrealistic in the number of exciting events that happen every evening but realistic in its portrayal of the roles of different healthcare professionals and the techniques they use. Someone who has never been to an accident and emergency department, and who doesn't have healthcare professionals among their friends, may believe that the representation is wholly realistic even when it isn't.

In the 1950s and 1960s, things were rosy in the medical drama. Over the past two decades, hospital and medical dramas have become more realistic and gritty. They show the effects of cutbacks, failed treatments, fallible and even culpable professionals. The American series *ER* uses a mix of actors and real-life professionals. Such changes of representation may reflect alterations in the real world. They are also a shift in media representation — away from portraying the healthcare professionals and services we would like to have and towards portraying those we actually have (Karpf, 1988). The changes also reflect the extent to which the media now penetrate people's lives. TV shows film of atrocities in Rwanda or the inside of orphanages and mental institutions in China and Romania. Newspapers carry pictures of Bosnian concentration camps on their front pages. We cannot pretend these things don't exist and the media amplify this load of knowledge that society carries, mainly in their news and feature programmes.

But the job of fictional programmes is also to entertain, even if their content is violent or shocking. There are still, however, some representations of the cosy and glamorous type, which appeal to some viewers. The series *Dangerfield* presented a heroic doctor who is always right, pursuing a relationship with a

'Four out of five of our panellists [all nurses] had watched [*Casualty*], and around 40% felt it gave an accurate portrayal of what was going on in the NHS. Few thought it was biased against the government.'

Nursing Times (1987) Vox pop. Media casualty? *Nursing Times* 83 (4): 22.

Here are some questions you might want to discuss with colleagues or others in your tutor/counsellor group:

- How accurately is the healthcare setting you work in represented on television, in dramas and factual reporting?

- Which sorts of things are represented realistically, and which sorts are glamorised, made more dramatic, or shown to be worse than they are?

- What effect do you think this misrepresentation has on patient/clients and their expectations of the service they get?

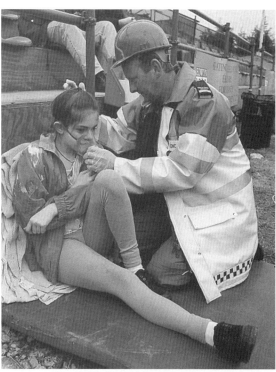

To the rescue : is this what it's really like?

glamorous woman doctor and doing good in his community. The return of *Dr Finlay's Casebook* to the screen showed that there is still a following for the reassuring view of the medical profession. At the other end of the spectrum, series about cuts and in-fighting in hospitals and the dark, disturbing portrayal of a psychologist in *Cracker* show an appetite for a more gritty fiction. The conventions of the genre are different, but is it more real?

Blurring the boundaries

Factual accounts of health care come in several forms: news, documentaries and 'real life' footage, such as *Hospital Watch*. Viewers are asked to believe that what they see is true, but they don't have to accept the claim at face value. There is, of necessity, selection and editing: these programmes cannot broadcast everything that happens in a hospital; producers have to pick the events and procedures that they think are interesting, or representative, or that fit the models of hospital representation and healthcare coverage they are used to.

Series such as *999* which re-enact rescues by paramedics and others working in the emergency services have started to blur the distinction between fact and fiction. Documentaries that include re-enactments of real events do much the same. Viewers are asked to believe that what they see is a representation of what really happened, but it is not a recording of the actual events. It is a model that requires sophisticated reception on the part of the viewer; perhaps it is not surprising if some viewers are unable to see the distinction between fiction and fact clearly, because some of the boundaries have been blurred.

'They wanted to see some people who were going to stay in the hospital until they died. I wanted to show them how we were treating patients so that they could recover and be discharged. They didn't want to see that. It wasn't how they thought of a geriatric ward.'

A consultant geriatrician whose hospital was featured in *Hospital Watch*.

'The newspaper is of necessity something of a monopoly, and its first duty is to shun the temptations of monopoly. Its primary office is the gathering of news. At the peril of its soul it must see that the supply is not tainted. Neither in what it gives, nor in what it does not give, nor in the mode of presentation, must the unclouded face of truth suffer wrong.'

Snow, C.P. (1964) *The Two Cultures and the Scientific Revolution.* Cambridge: Cambridge University Press.

What do people who are not healthcare professionals believe when they see scenes like those in *999* enacted on television? They have to make complex judgements about which bits are 'true' and which bits matter. Maybe the producer's judgement of what matters doesn't match the opinion of healthcare professionals, or those viewing the programme.

You might want to investigate these issues as part of your assessment for the unit. For example, you could take a programme or series, find out how healthcare professionals and non-professionals react to it and compare their reactions. Your tutor/counsellor will be able to help you design a suitable method for doing this sort of survey.

'Every news story should, without sacrifice of probity or responsibility, display the attributes of fiction, of drama.'

Reuven Frank, quoted in Hartley (1982) *Understanding News.* London: Methuen. (Reprinted 1988, Routledge, London.)

Who gets heard?

Are voices in the media representative of society? It used to be said that the powerful, wealthy and well-educated have privileged access to the media and that their voices are heard more loudly: they can put issues on the agenda and get their opinions heard by policy-makers and the public, while the poor, elderly and unemployed generally don't have a voice and are under-represented in media coverage and are rarely consulted or canvassed for information or their views. When they do get a hearing, it is believed, it is generally because the privileged choose to approach them, not because they successfully access the channels of information on their own.

But how biased is this view? Channel 4 commissions programmes for various cultures, ages and social groups. The *Sun* and the *Mirror* would say ordinary people write and speak in their pages. Professional journals such as *Nursing Times* talk to their readers all the time and also give them the opportunity to talk in their own voices. They 'provide a marvellous forum for novice writers to air their views and to develop their writing and critical abilities'; they also 'have the potential to influence the perceptions of clients, managers and politicians about current professional developments, problems and concerns' (Smith, 1996).

However, it is true that wealthy people provide financial support to the press and that a paper's editorial line can reflect the opinions and prejudices of the proprietor as much as its editorial staff.

Concentration of power

Power in the media may be concentrated in a relatively small group of people, as it is in other walks of life. These people have friends in other professions and in government. They give each other media exposure and further each other's interests in their own areas of influence. As long as power and influence are concentrated in a privileged group, they will stay there. But the bastion of media power is not impregnable. For instance, through persistent lobbying, disabled groups have gained a voice. There are now programmes for disabled viewers and listeners, and the needs of disabled people are taken seriously by policy-makers. Women have now gained positions of power and responsibility in publishing, TV and radio that go well beyond the traditional areas of women's magazines and programmes related to the home. Many high-

---

'Outside the nursing journals, nurses and, indeed, the RCN, find it very difficult to get media attention for good news about nursing...It is rare to see nurses interviewed or reported as experts in a field of care. It is highly unusual to find a nurse explaining to the public the advantages of a new form of care or treatment or spreading the good news about a hospital or clinic.'

Hancock, C. (1991) Blowing the trumpet. *Nursing Times* 87: 34: 26-8.

This was in 1991. How much have things changed? Could Christine Hancock make the same comments today, in your view?

'To inform, to discuss, to mirror, to bind, to campaign, to challenge, to entertain, to judge — these are the important functions of the media in any free country.'

Curran, J. and Seaton, J. (1991) *Power Without Responsibility. The press and broadcasting in Britain* (4th edition). London: Routledge.

Individuals can affect media coverage in several ways, though they are more likely to be heard if they can speak through an organisation. If you or one of your patients or clients had an experience or wanted to raise an issue which you think warrants wider public exposure, you could:

- Contact the news desk of a paper, television or radio station
- Write a letter to a local or national paper
- Contact a consumer programme
- Contact the health editor of a publication, or the health correspondent of a television or radio channel to suggest a topic which could be covered.

Section 5 contains advice on communicating with the media and getting your case across in a way which will maximise the chances of its being taken up and covered as you would wish.

profile news reporters and presenters are women, including foreign correspondents reporting from a war zone.

The voices of health care

In the past, when reporters wanted a quotation from a healthcare professional on an aspect of government policy, they almost always approached a doctor or academic, rarely a nurse or other healthcare professional unless the issue was specifically related to that profession. The assumption that doctors speak with more authority and will be better regarded by the public, even though in some cases the experience and insight of a different healthcare professional may be more relevant, is less pervasive today. Nowadays, journalists are just as likely to ask for the views of the general secretary of the Royal College of Nursing. The voice of senior medical professionals — doctors, surgeons and consultants — is no longer always needed to legitimate medical issues.

Even so, the voice of an organisation such as the British Medical Association (BMA) is still powerful, partly because doctors, surgeons and consultants are respected and powerful in their own right. In December 1987, 1200 senior

doctors and professors signed a petition condemning NHS cuts. Before this, complaints about bed cuts and reduced funding were not treated as seriously or extensively by the media. After the BMA intervention, cutbacks became a more legitimate issue for media coverage, and have remained so.

'In 1987 the Conservative party had 43% of the vote, but 72% of national daily newspaper circulation.'

Curran, J. and Seaton, J. (1991) ibid.

In January 1996, the Home Office was forced to review regulations which allowed women prisoners in the later stages of pregnancy and in labour to be shackled during hospital visits.

The procedure had been introduced in 1995 when some male prisoners had made attempts to escape from custody during outside visits. The improbability of a woman in labour attempting to escape clearly wasn't taken into account.

Midwives had on several occasions objected to the shackling of women in labour, but the affair only became a national scandal after the friend of a woman prisoner smuggled a video camera into a hospital room and filmed secretly. Public outcry followed the revelation of the procedure and, in a matter of days, the Home Office gave way, entirely as the result of media exposure.

On February 4, 1988, the *Guardian* devoted a page to articles about the nurses' day of action the previous day. One article on the page was entitled 'Doctors call for immediate injection of cash to revive crumbling service' and related how the BMA has asked for £1,500m to be invested in the NHS.

Do you think the *Guardian* editor felt that the doctors' demand legitimised the nurses' claims, and that their case wasn't strong enough alone? Does this sort of thing happen often, in your experience? Look through some of the healthcare stories you collect during your work on this book. Who is quoted in the articles? You might like to perform a proper quantitative study as a larger piece of research, either for your assessment on this unit or as an enquiry topic for the core unit, *Enquiring into Healthcare Practice*.

Whose viewpoint?

When people look at a painting or a photograph, they are engaged in an act of interpretation at several levels, conscious and unconscious. At one and the same time they may be:

- Consciously working out what the picture 'shows'
- Responding unconsciously to its sensorimotor impact
- Bringing to bear on the interpretation — in a semi-conscious way — what they already know about the artist or the subject.

Even with all this interpretation going on, they may get drawn in and become unaware that a point of view is imposed on them as a viewer. Similarly, when people read a press report, or watch a television broadcast, it is easy to get drawn in and forget that there is a point of view in there.

A photograph is taken from a particular position, by a photographer looking in a particular direction; the choice of position, camera angle and what is included in the shot make up the picture and colour our interpretation of the event recorded. Artists choose their subject and materials, their position in the scene and the size of the painting; a commissioned portrait for public display will differ from a lover's private picture, or a miniature. The same is true of a written or broadcast report. A point of view influences:

- The choice and order of words
- The angle the reporter takes on the story
- The decision to include the story in a publication or programme and where to place it in the 'flow' — what McLuhan (1964) called 'a deliberate artistic aim in the placing and management of news'.

The effects of the creator's point of view are easier to see in a picture, but are just as significant in a written or broadcast account of an event or story. Uncritical readers, listeners and viewers may be unaware of the point of view of the writer or broadcaster, or pay little attention to it. Developing an awareness of this is a first step in gaining greater insight into how the media works on us.

Realistic perspective and reality

A significant development in Western art in the 14th and 15th centuries was the emergence of a perspective view, reputedly invented (or rediscovered) by Filippo Brunelleschi (1377–1446). This is now taken as the norm for

---

'Realism is plausible not because it reflects the world, but because it is constructed out of what is (discursively) familiar.'

Belsey, C. (1980) *Critical Practice*. London: Methuen.

'Perspective is nothing else than seeing a place behind a sheet of glass, smooth and quite transparent, on the surface of which all the things may be marked that are behind this glass...Of several bodies, all equally large and equally distant, that which is most brightly illuminated will appear to the eye nearest and largest.'

Richter, A. (ed.) (1977). *Selections from the Notebooks of Leonardo da Vinci*. Oxford: Oxford University Press.

How 'realistic' are the pictures on the opposite page? Think about what they aim to convey and how successful they are in doing so.

There is an interesting discussion of how we look at and understand images, including a critique of the symbolism used in Hans Holbein the Younger's painting 'The Ambassadors' (pictured centre opposite), in:

Berger, G. (1990) *Ways of Seeing*. Harmondsworth: Penguin Books.

The construction of meaning by the interaction of viewer/reader and picture/text is a recurring theme in this book. Bear it in mind as you analyse media representations. You could build up a picture in your portfolio of what you bring to the media — your prejudices, emotions, experience — and how these contribute to the meanings you find or construct.

In a 'realistic' perspective view, we lose sight of the artist or photographer unless they provide a reminder of their presence. In the Velázquez painting 'Las Meninas' (1656), the artist portrays himself, apparently painting the king and queen reflected in the mirror. His presence reminds us we are looking at a portrait for which real people are sitting. We become aware of the painting as artifice, a staged event executed over time. We see its process, not just the finished and static image usually seen in a portrait.

representational works of art, yet it was not widely used before the 14th century and is not used by all cultures today.

A perspective view represents a scene as it is perceived by a single viewer in a single position at one moment in time. It has a vanishing point — the point where lines which are parallel appear to meet as you look at the scene. In a perspective view, distant objects look comparatively smaller than objects close to the viewer (or in the foreground of the picture). The objects are not really smaller, but they look smaller: a perspective view shows things as they appear to be. Perspective represents a single viewpoint.

We tend to be aware of perspective in paintings only when it is distorted or ignored. Mediaeval paintings often depict the most important elements in the scene as the largest, or put them in the foreground regardless of their real position. The size and position of an object reflects its importance. Cubist images may offer several views or facets of the same object or scene within a single picture, conveying the multiple viewpoints that are excluded by perspective. A child's picture may show no

awareness of perspective, or the relative sizes of objects, but reflect the child's perception of the importance or attractiveness of different elements — or even just that they are detailed and difficult to draw small.

These alternative types of view can make us think about what constitutes reality. Is it just what we see, or is it the meaning of what we see? Meaning comes also from what we bring to a picture or piece of text — how we interpret something depends on our own view of the world and the links we make between things. These are useful things to remember when learning to look critically at media representations of reality.

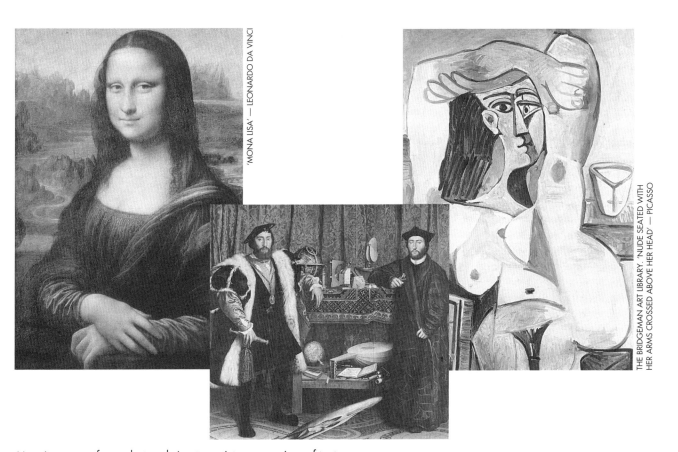

'MONA LISA' — LEONARDO DA VINCI

THE BRIDGEMAN ART LIBRARY. 'NUDE SEATED WITH HER ARMS CROSSED ABOVE HER HEAD' — PICASSO

Meaning comes from what we bring to a picture or a piece of text

Perspectives in media images

When you watch a broadcast or look at a photograph in a newspaper or magazine, it is revealing to think about the point of view or perspective it is promoting. Camera angle, lighting, the background, the positions of the people and all elements of the picture's composition contribute to its meaning and effect. Its relationship to other images or text can also add to or alter the meaning the picture would have if looked at in isolation.

Reading images

In the adjacent column are two photographs of a politician. One shows her in a casual pose and clothes, the other in formal dress. In one she is with her family, in the other she is with other politicians. It would not be necessary to read the accompanying news report to guess the type of article each picture illustrates. The first says 'family matters' or 'positive PR job'; the second supports a story about official business.

Body language and dress codes are both ways of creating an image. Politicians use them skilfully — they are trained to know what they will look like when a camera is pointed at them. Media pictures often use a sort of iconographic shorthand. Particular images call up resonances

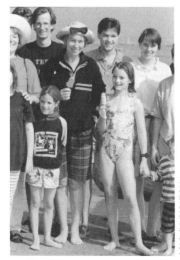

Unofficial business

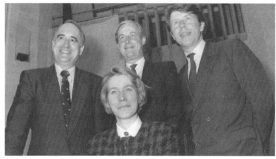

Official business

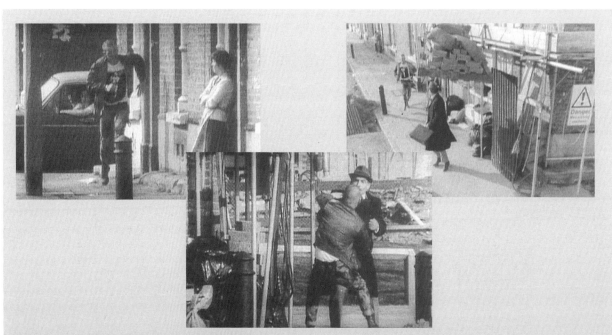

What is included in a picture helps to define its meaning. This series of images is from a television advertisement for the *Guardian*. The scene in the centre looks like a mugging — the dress and appearance of the man endorse this reading. We may make assumptions about people based on factors like these. In fact the man in the bomber jacket is saving the old man from a potential accident (centre picture). The sequence makes us analyse our assumptions about people as well as think about how selectivity can change the meaning of a picture.

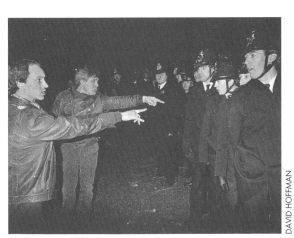

Is anyone breaking the law?

DAVID HOFFMAN

and connotations that confer meaning without verbal commentary. There is an assumption that people looking at it will know the code and will read the picture as the originator intended it to be read — although they might not. The unwritten code in the photograph above is that the workers, who are shown opposing the police, are law-breakers (whether or not they actually are breaking the law). The picture imposes an interpretation of the situation: it is not the only interpretation, but it may be hard to resist. What did you think when you first looked at the photograph?

Pictures in context

The position of images on a page in relation to other pictures and text, or their place in a broadcast sequence, also adds to their meaning. The juxtaposition of a semi-nude model with a story about a sex crime is intended to be titillating, but many people will find it a cheap and distasteful abuse of the news story. Some will be excited by the picture and the story and may find that both have more impact because they are presented together.

Myra Hindley, the Moors murderer (below left), is made to look 'monstrous' by choosing a sullen, serious and unflattering photo. The more natural portrait beneath it conveys a more disturbing message when you know who it is — she looks 'normal' and could be anyone. There is more about images in the media on pages 80–83.

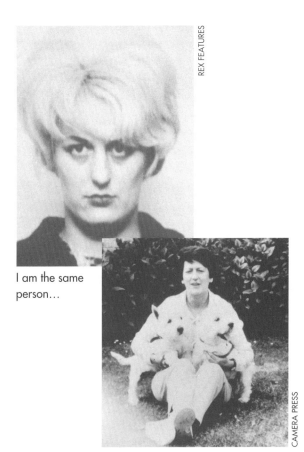

I am the same person...

...or not?

REX FEATURES / CAMERA PRESS

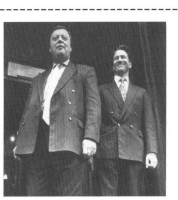

THE INDEPENDENT

What impression does this photograph of politicians Michael Portillo and Kenneth Clarke produce? Ask two or three other people and work out how the photograph achieves its intended effect.

'I am sometimes accused by my peers of printing my pictures too dark. All I can say is that it goes with the mood of melancholy that is induced by witnessing at close quarters such intractable situations of conflict and joylessness.'
McCullin, D. (1994) *Sleeping with Ghosts: A life's work in photography*. London: Jonathan Cape.

Different voices

All people have their own recognisable range of voices. Journalists adopt a particular voice when writing or broadcasting to suit their audience and to communicate a slant on the story. The voice helps to convey a point of view. Part of being a critical reader is to become aware of this. In some cases, the voice may be distinctive and it is easy to hear the voice of the writer. In other cases an individual voice may not be so recognisable. It takes practice to 'hear' the voice and to make allowances for it in the interpretation.

Actual voices heard on radio and TV can be powerful. It is not always easy to focus critical attention on what someone is saying if the person has a persuasive voice. Conversely, the absence of a voice may also be powerful. Many stars of the silent movies became has-beens when they started to speak in films because their audiences were disappointed with the sound of their voices. Some of the power of media figures such as Gerry Adams, leader of Sinn Fein, may have come from the fact that they were banned from speaking on TV.

What's in a word?

Television and radio news has a set of standards or beliefs shared by many or most viewers or listeners. This influences the choice of words and gives the story an angle or an interpretation which may be hard to detect.

On November 4, 1995, the Israeli prime minister, Yitzhak Rabin, was shot dead by a gunman. Most newspaper and television reports said that he had been assassinated. But one radio report mentioned the 'murder' of Rabin. This word colours the story differently. An assassination is assumed to have a political motive. Our expectations are overturned and our understanding of the event challenged by the choice of the word 'murder', which is generally used in a different sphere of reference. Thus some words have associations which form part of their meaning. The 'war' in the Falklands defined the terms of Britain's opposition to Argentina, but the 'troubles' in Northern Ireland are not described as 'war'. A possible interpretation is that the word 'war' would give the 'troubles' a status that the British government does not want to recognise.

Reports often contain clues that indicate whether the piece is presented as a point of view or as fact:

- Phrases such as 'I think', or 'I believe' are a clear indication that it is the author's point of view that is being explained.

- Use of the passive voice — 'it is believed that', 'it is thought that' — suggests that everyone agrees and it is not just an opinion. But does everyone really agree?

- Statements that present something as a fact — '50% of women are larger than size 14' — do not invite examination. Such statements have an air of authority and we don't automatically question them. But should we?

- Quoting an authoritative voice or source is often used as a means of validating a statement. But shouldn't we question the authority of the quotation?

There is more on the way people communicate, using words and other forms of language, including body language, in Section 4 of the unit entitled *Professional Relationships: Influences on health care*.

'Terrorism: a policy intended to strike with terror those against whom it is adopted; the employment of methods of intimidation.'

Oxford English Dictionary. Oxford: Oxford University Press, 1971.

There they were, as if our memory hatched them,
As if the unquiet founders walked again:
Two young men with rifles on the hill,
Profane and bracing as their instruments.
Who's sorry for our trouble?
Seamus Heaney (1979) Triptych: After a Killing. In: *Field Work*. London: Faber.

The connotations of a word affect how people accept a news story, and how the event is categorised. Reporters or newspaper sub-editors may choose one word in preference to alternatives to convey meaning more precisely; but they may also choose a particular word for its connotations and the way it promotes the chosen interpretation of events. For example, IRA acts of violence are commonly called terrorism in this country. This assumes a shared moral and political stance opposed to the IRA and its methods. In fact, there may be many people who support the aims espoused by the IRA but reject and abhor its methods. Acts similar in kind perpetrated by groups that we may be expected to support might be described instead as the political activism or armed struggle of guerrilla fighters. Hartley (1982) points out that a reporter is unlikely to say 'terrorists liberated' because the words 'terrorist' and 'liberate' come from two opposing discourses — we approve of liberation, but disapprove of terrorism.

Who's listening?

Meaning depends partly on the connotations and resonance of the chosen words. But it also depends on who is listening. Individuals speak differently to different audiences, and so do the media. At one level, a specialist publication or programme uses the special vocabulary (jargon) that its intended audience will understand and expect. This use of jargon reinforces the identity of the audience and may exclude those who do not understand it. At another level, a newspaper chooses its language to suit the readership it has, or wishes to attract. It usually endorses its readers' view of themselves by reflecting their value system. So the *Sun's* characteristic headlines are colloquial, laddish and irreverently humorous, while the serious broadsheets are restrained and generally less emotive.

The most important part of meaning is that people bring their own experiences and value systems to bear on interpreting an image or a report. If something conflicts with their value system, they may spot it and dismiss the report. Newspapers may attempt to change value systems by careful choice of presentation. Some people may accept the presented version and the news may help to re-mould their views. But this does not always happen — people are inclined to stick with the lessons of their own accumulated experience.

In the healthcare professions, people tend to work alongside colleagues and talk to each other, for example in breaks or in the staff room. Listen to what they say in these off-duty moments. If you hear them telling a story to two different people or voicing an opinion to different groups, notice how the 'voice' changes.

- How do people's voices come across?
- How do they vary their accounts to meet the expectations of their different audiences?
- What words or expressions did they use for one audience, but not the other?

See if you can catch yourself out doing this sort of thing. It shows how flexible and creative people are with language!

On November 3, 1995, a local paper ran the headline: 'Medics plan pioneer op'. The story goes on to describe how cells from aborted fetuses may be used in an attempt to reverse brain damage in patients with Huntington's disease. There is clearly an ethics issue to be considered. The report acknowledges this: 'Anti-abortion organisations condemned the move. A spokesman for LIFE...said similar operations had been carried out elsewhere to combat Parkinson's disease and had produced no long-term benefits. However...'

What do the 'However' and the cheery headline say about the newspaper's stance in relation to the new medical technique?

The language used about illness directs our responses to it and affects the perceptions of both sufferers and society in general. This theme is explored in:

Sontag, S. (1991) *Illness as Metaphor*. London: Penguin.

Subjectivity and objectivity

Readers, listeners and viewers may expect objectivity from programmes and publications which set themselves up as deliverers of news or documentary material but not from those that overtly campaign on behalf of a cause or take sides over an issue. But is it possible to have an objective account of events or issues in the media?

'Objective' reporting

Some publications and television and radio programmes present themselves as unbiased sources giving objective coverage. But how objective are they really? Objectivity can be compromised by:

- The mode of expression and manner of presentation
- The selection of material to include or exclude
- The degree of prominence given to different elements or viewpoints.

Reporters may select to create as little bias as possible, or to be deliberately controversial. Neutrality has its own pitfalls: words and phrases can become platitudes and lose real meaning; the way 'facts' are presented can become stylised and follow the same conventions.

Any report is, of necessity, a partial relation and interpretation of events. The choice of words, images and method of presentation involves some degree of selection and some level of interpretation. A mediated event — one we do not experience directly — is interpreted both by the teller and the listener. Even an event experienced directly is interpreted as we make sense of it; perception itself is an act of interpretation.

Subjective reports

Subjectivity is the acknowledged expression of an individual's or group's point of view. Common examples in the media are:

- The editorial or comment column in a newspaper or magazine
- A named columnist writing in a newspaper, or a regular contributor's column in a magazine
- The TV chat show or discussion programme in which members of the public share and discuss their views and experiences
- Readers' letters in a newspaper or magazine
- Personal views of the type produced by the *Video Nation* series — individuals' records of their daily lives made with a video camera and broadcast without editorial comment.

Which publications and programmes do you trust to be objective? Watch or read them critically for a while and see if you can uncover a hidden agenda, or how they work to promote a viewpoint. Use your learning journal to keep a record or diary of what you find.

The public gets what the public wants.

The public wants what the public gets.

And I don't care what this society wants,

I'm going underground...

Going Underground. Words from a song by The Jam, 1980

'The *Independent*: it is – are you?'

Advertising for the newly-launched *Independent* stressed its impartiality, clearly expecting this to be an attractive feature.

Why would the slogan not work if it said 'we are – are you'?

'The BBC takes it for granted that the parliamentary democracy evolved in this country is a work of national genius to be upheld and preserved...'

'...a newspaper has a point of view and a place on the political spectrum. The BBC has none.'

BBC (1976) *The Task of Broadcasting News.* London: BBC Publications.

These two statements are from the same programme. How are they contradictory?

If the first view represented the BBC's position, could the BBC present objective reports if there were a civil war in the UK attempting to overthrow parliamentary democracy?

An editorial is a commentary on the issues covered in the news reporting or in other features. It has the authority of the publication behind it and normally reflects the views held by readers, although it may also challenge them. Named columnists have a licence to express their own opinions, which may not wholly reflect those of the publication; they tend to have distinctive opinions and colourful personalities. Readers expect to see a personal viewpoint, and accept that it will be strongly held and powerfully expressed. Moreover, they will respond to individual articles and the balance of coverage. They may also report their personal experiences.

On television, public forum shows such as *Kilroy* invite people to share their experiences and views, often on issues related to health care such as cosmetic surgery, caring for elderly relatives, psychiatric problems and coping with cancer. The aim of these programmes is to show different voices and sources of experience; they rarely make judgements.

Responses to reporting

People tend to respond differently to overtly subjective reporting and to reports that are presented as objective. News reports may combine objective and subjective accounts of events. For example, articles in magazines on healthcare issues often use subjective case histories to back up the factual reporting.

How they are read depends on how much the reader knows. Healthcare professionals may be more able to decide whether a health-related story is accurate or believable than people who do not have that knowledge and experience.

There may be differences in emotional and rational responses to objective and subjective reporting and they stimulate different kinds of insight or response. If you hear about a plane crash, you will understand rationally the fact that 273 people have been killed. But what can bring the event home, or give a context for understanding it, may be a detail: one passenger was travelling to meet up with a long-lost brother, or a couple on the flight were on their honeymoon. Sometimes, objective reports may produce a distanced response through the use of technical or medical language.

The following is part of an editorial from a national daily newspaper on January 8, 1996.

'....not before time, the nursing profession is being opened up to market forces. In a pioneering move, an Essex hospital trust is offering nurses with scarce skills a golden hello of up to £2,000...

'As competition for specialised nurses pushes up their value, so more young women and men should find it worth their while to undergo the extra training required. But most people may only begin to believe in the benign effects of the internal market with the National Health Service when it remedies both the glut of managers and the dearth of key nurses.'

What type of reader do you think this paper believes it is addressing?

What values are implicit in the editorial?

Section 3 of the unit entitled *Professional Relationships: Influences on health care* has more on people's values and the process of socialisation that creates them.

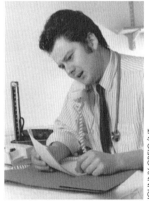

JOHNNY GREIG/NT

The 'problem page' is a common way of covering health care and emotional issues in magazines and newspapers. Look at the photograph above of a doctor who answers health questions on the problem page.

What can you say about his appearance, his body position and expression?

What does his appearance tell you about this magazine's readers' expectations of a doctor?

Do you think it is possible to predict his viewpoint on some issues from his appearance and from what you know of this type of article?

Choosing the news

What makes a news story? An event or issue has to be 'newsworthy' to be reported. It also helps if it can be interpreted to fit in with the established framework for news reporting.

Events tend to be more newsworthy than issues. So events are often used as a 'peg' for a story about issues. The closure of an accident and emergency department may be the peg for a story about cuts in the health service, or an industrial dispute may be the peg for a story about the power of unions. Cuts in the health service and economic depression don't usually have enough news value without the peg to make them topical. Once an event has passed it is no longer newsworthy, and the 24-hour cycle of news gathering means that reporters move on to something else. Only further impact can keep an event in the news. Even then it may not be covered, unless the new development is not sufficiently arresting or sensational.

Dominant ideology

Is there a set of standards and views which informs and determines news coverage?

Stories may be selected according to whether they support and endorse common media stereotypes. For example, news stories about health care may focus on high-profile modern medicine, home-based care, alternative therapies or how lifestyle affects health. A 'good news' story may feature a medical breakthrough, or an encouraging report on care or waiting lists. A 'bad news' story may be about an epidemic or cut-backs in the health service. Researchers who support the 'dominant ideology' thesis think that because almost all reports are of this type, the public's view of health provision tends to be disproportionately focused on these issues (Herman and Chomsky, 1988).

You may find evidence of some form of dominant ideology yourself. But media culture is very often more diverse and less homogeneous than this suggests. What about the alternatives? For example, a programme like *Woman's Hour* does a lot on alternative therapies, and women's magazines often pick on topics such as home births, breast versus bottle feeding and other issues challenging received wisdom.

Parkin (1982) has identified three alternative ways in which a dominant ideology may be interpreted. People may accept the message (the dominant code), partially resist it (negotiated

---

Are the criteria for news selection in tune with people's desires and expectations? Look through a newspaper and discuss with colleagues or others in your tutor/counsellor group whether you are interested in the topics covered. Do people always want to read about the royal family?

When the IRA bombing of Canary Wharf in February 1996 prevented printing of the *Guardian* in London, the paper decided to put as much of its coverage as possible on its on-line paper on the World Wide Web. The editor decided to change the main headline at 2 am, only minutes before the electronic version was made available to the public – this couldn't have happened with a printed paper.

'The function of a daily news service is not simply the continuous up to the minute monitoring, processing and defining of immediate national and international news events. It also serves to define the currency and topicality of events and issues for current affairs programmes.'

Scannell, P. (1979) The social eye of television 1946-1955. In: *Media, Culture and Society* 1(1): 97-106.

Collect several daily papers and monitor the television and radio news for a day. You will probably find many of the same stories covered in each.

Why do you think the news stories were chosen?

Are the different papers and broadcast media using the same criteria to determine newsworthiness?

How are the stories treated differently?

decoding) or fully refuse it (oppositional code). For example, imagine the government were to end the exemption from prescription charges for all pregnant women and introduce selective exemption based on means testing instead. Three responses might be:
- Agree it's a good idea as it will save money for other healthcare provision and won't disadvantage women who can't afford to pay
- Agree that it will save money, but have reservations — some people may not understand the system and will pay when they don't have to, or the limits may not be appropriately set
- Reject the idea completely — some women who fail the means test may not pay for medicines they need.

History of a news story
Leah Betts was admitted to hospital early on November 12, 1995, after taking Ecstasy. She suffered respiratory arrest and went into a coma. She died on November 17. Her father and step-mother talked to the press and allowed her picture to be used in the hope of warning other teenagers against drug misuse. The following headlines are taken from the Electronic *Telegraph*, a news service on the World Wide

Web (http://www.telegraph.co.uk). They tell their own fascinating story about how the media choose news.

November 14, 1995: 'Hope fades for Ecstasy drug victim'.
Leah Betts was still in a coma.

November 16: 'Doctors treating a girl in a coma after she took a contaminated Ecstasy tablet at her 18th birthday party said last night there was a "significant chance" she would die'.
It turned out later that the tablet Leah had taken was pure.

November 17: 'Parents speak out as Ecstasy girl dies'.

November 23: 'Nightclub pair sought over Leah's death'.

February 1, 1996: 'Leah had taken Ecstasy before, inquest told'.

February 5: 'Leah's photo hijacked to back Ecstasy'.

March 6: 'Leah's liver was sent abroad because of a bed shortage'.

Jonathan Street, a public relations professional specialising in NHS news, comments on the Leah Betts story: 'I got a call from the hospital where she was on a ventilator on the Sunday night. Already the police were making the news agenda because her father was an ex-policeman. There was much comment later, when the Poisons Unit at Guy's established that it was the water that killed her, about media "over-reaction". In my view they had no choice... there was no way that anyone could wait for the pathology report.'

This view was not shared by everyone:

'If [Leah's] death had been pushed in less simple terms, to include her way of death, perhaps it would have prevented Helen Cousins falling into a coma from drinking seven litres of water after taking Ecstasy two months later.'

Walter, N. (1996) Dead women who suit the news agenda. *Guardian*, January 18, 1996.

These books have useful material on news values and the meaning of the news:

Hartley, J. *Understanding News*. London: Methuen. (Reprinted 1988, Routledge, London.)

Glasgow Media Group (1976) *Bad News*. London: Routledge.

Glasgow Media Group (1980) *More Bad News*. London: Routledge.

Whitaker, B. (1981) *News Limited: Why you can't read all about it*. London: Minority Press Group.

The whole truth and nothing but the truth?

Sometimes it may not greatly matter to most readers whether a report is true or not; for example, if a gossip column reports an actress having an affair. At other times they expect the facts to be accurate. But it may be difficult to judge what is true, even in apparently simple cases such as the two headlines that follow:

'The government reports an unemployment figure of 2.5 million.'
This looks authoritative, but as with all statistics the figure quoted depends on the method of counting. The number of unemployed can be reduced by counting only those who have been out of work for more than six weeks, are registered as available for work and who are currently claiming benefit. The figure can be increased by including all people who are not in work, whether or not they are looking for work or want to work. The actual number of people who consider themselves unemployed — who want to work and don't have a job — lies somewhere in between. A truer statement would be: 'Using its method of calculating the figures, the government estimates that unemployment is currently 2.5 million.' (See pages 76-77 for more on the presentation of statistics in the media.)

'The average waiting time for a hip replacement operation is nine months.'
A statement like this may also be misleading. In general, waiting times are calculated from the point at which a patient is accepted on the waiting list by a consultant. This account gives no indication that patients may need to wait several months to see a consultant, even though their GP may have told them they need a hip replacement operation. A truer statement would be: 'The average delay between seeing a consultant and having a hip replacement operation is nine months.'

Bald statements like these headlines can disguise the complexity of the issues underneath. For example, a report which took seriously the debate about waiting lists would need to look at what people expect — they may not mind waiting longer if they get effective care when they do see the specialist. Also, some waiting lists may have to be longer for complex reasons which are not reflected in targets like these.

'What is truth?' said jesting Pilate; and would not stay for an answer.

Francis Bacon (1994) Of truth. In: *Essays.* London: Everyman Series, J.M. Dent.

'I'm worried about Emma. She should be doing better at school.'

'The trouble with him is that he's not romantic enough.'

Could you live outside the influence of the media? How does it impinge on the way you bring up children or relate to your partner? Take a notebook with you one day when you are not at work and jot down every time you become aware that you are interacting with the media in any way.

Look back at your notes at the end of the day. What do you see?

'Journalists say a thing that they know isn't true, in the hope that if they keep on saying it long enough it will be true.'

Arnold Bennett: *The Title*, Act II.

'I hesitate to say what the functions of the modern journalist may be; but I imagine that they do not exclude the intelligent anticipation of facts even before they occur.'

Lord Curzon of Kedleston. Speech in the House of Commons, March 29, 1898.

Do you think the press deserves to be widely disbelieved?

Why do people watch television news and read the newspapers if they don't believe they will get the true story?

Is it a journalist's job to report or to educate?

News and current affairs deal in theories, interpretations, unfinished research and partial reports. There may be clues to the status of the information presented, which a critical reader or viewer will pick up. Phrases such as 'researchers believe they have uncovered...' or 'reports are emerging of a massacre...' indicate that we are not getting verified fact. When a report does get something completely wrong, there may sometimes be an apology or retraction. But these usually have little impact and are given little prominence, as those who have successfully claimed libel against the newspapers have found. As healthcare and medical reporting often involves unfamiliar science, there is extra potential for getting it wrong — and what happens if people do not have the knowledge to spot the errors (Dixon, 1994)?

Case study

On November 17, 1994, Central TV's *Cook Report* ran the first of two reports entitled 'The Cot-Death Poisonings'. The reports claimed that a fire retardant chemical used in cot mattresses could in some circumstances emit a toxic substance which might poison babies. They included statistics from specially commissioned tests, the findings of which were tentative but which suggested a link which should be investigated.

Morning television programmes on the day the first *Cook Report* was due to be broadcast covered the findings of the report. Public interest was immediate and intense. Reaction from the establishment was swift and adverse. Other bodies researching the issues denounced the report's findings and methods. A few days after the first report was broadcast, an expert speaking on BBC TV's *Good Morning* programme said that the findings of the report had been largely discredited, even though no further research had been carried out at this point. Many worried parents could not tell what was 'true' from the television coverage. Were babies at risk from a source they previously had not considered? Or was it 'true' that the report was inaccurate? If it was inaccurate was it completely 'untrue'; that is, was there no risk to babies from their mattresses?

Patients 'nursed in recovery area'

Quotation marks are often used in headlines to indicate that something is an allegation and may not be true. They also flag phraseology as not being the publication's own words or view. Other devices can be used to hide sources or flag off-the-record remarks:

'Sources close to... — this means someone's assistant or colleague.

'A close friend of ...' — the person themselves, but the remark is not attributable.

'Friends of' — almost anyone who knows the person and is prepared to make a remark that is not attributable.

'Journals such as *The Lancet*, *BMJ*, *Nature*, *Science*, *JAMA* and *NEJM* have high credibility by virtue of the peer-review system... Richard Smith, editor of *BMJ*, maintains that only 5% of what these and other peer-reviewed journals publish is credible, the rest being "rubbish".'
Pini, P. (1995) Media wars. *The Lancet* 346: 1683.

This is a highly contentious statement. How could you check its accuracy? Discuss with others in your tutor/counsellor group how you could establish the level of credibility in articles published in reputable journals. You may decide to carry out a critique of a number of articles relating to your professional field as part of your assessment for this unit.

Frameworks and straitjackets

News reporting is easiest — though not necessarily best — if the reporter can slot a story into a predetermined framework. Since news reporting has to be concise and get the message across quickly, it uses a sort of shorthand which the consumer of news as well as the producers understand. If you look at newspapers or watch or listen to broadcast news, you will quickly spot formulas and structures that are used again and again. These affect the parts of the story that are covered, the choice of language and images and how the story is fitted in with others. Once the reporter, editor or producer has chosen the right framework for a particular story, the choice of images and language and its relation to other stories quickly falls into place. As with producing, so with receiving: the conventional frameworks are easily interpreted by the audience. They don't take much thought.

Models of healthcare reporting

Healthcare reporting has increased dramatically since the start of the 1980s (Entwhistle and Hancock-Beaulieu, 1992) and has developed its own frameworks. Once inside a framework, a story is assigned a particular type of significance and this is reinforced by the way it is presented. If it doesn't fit, it may be shoe-horned into a framework or abandoned altogether. The four main frameworks for healthcare reporting (Karpf, 1988) are:

- The medical model
- The consumer model
- The 'help-yourself' model
- The environmental model.

The medical model

The medical model focuses on the achievements of modern medicine and technology, and equates better health care with more spending on, and consumption of, healthcare services and medicine. It has a curative bias, puts doctors, consultants and surgeons in the foreground and is characterised by reporting of new developments in medicine and treatment, and stories of recovery and recuperation. The rhetoric of doctors 'battling' with disease, of patients 'saved' and of epidemics 'rampaging' and viruses 'attacking' gives drama to this coverage (Dixon, 1994).

The consumer model

The consumer's perspective in health care focuses on patients/clients, and their relationship with doctors and healthcare professionals. It may include patients' rights and experiences and has

---

Look at these extracts from a woman's magazine and a local paper in the light of the frameworks identified above.

How far do they fit into the models outlined?

Do they step outside the frameworks, or combine elements from different models?

'Beating heart disease
Eating an orange a day could reduce your risk of heart disease by 10 per cent. Researchers have found that high levels of vitamin C reduce the body's levels of fibrinogen — a protein which aids blood clotting and, in high levels, can increase the risk of heart disease.'

Options October 1995, p10

'When you are too poor to eat for two
As soon as a pregnancy test is positive, women are bombarded with advice on how to stay fit and healthy. High on the list is a balanced diet. But a report from two charities shows that for an increasing number of women, especially young ones, a healthy diet is off the menu because they cannot afford it...Bridy Speller, spokeswoman for the Thames Anglia region of NCH Action for Children said: "We know that the difficulties faced by pregnant women in eating a healthy, balanced diet aren't the result of lack of knowledge, but of poor material circumstances and low incomes."

Cambridge Evening News, November 21, 1995

In your view, does 'help yourself' healthcare reporting shift responsibility onto the individual or empower the individual? How useful do you find it in making sense of your own health problems? What effect does it have on your practice as a healthcare professional?

been given a focus in *The Patient's Charter*.

The help-yourself model
The recent explosion of interest in healthy living, diet and exercise has pushed the 'help yourself' school of reporting into the limelight. This takes the view that individuals can and should take charge of their own health. It focuses on preventive health care, with diet and exercise important cornerstones of the healthy living régime. This approach also picks up on the government agenda of people taking responsibility for themselves.

The environmental model
The environmental perspective focuses on how factors in the environment combine to affect people's health. This includes the role of poverty-induced poor diet, damaging working conditions, pollution, poor housing and other factors beyond the individual's control. Because of its political resonances and the large-scale social changes required to make any real difference, this perspective tends to receives less exposure in the mass media than the others.

Each of these perspectives links in some way to the political and social agendas reported in (and often amplified by) the media. The inter-relations may be subtle and paradoxical. For example, *The Patient's Charter* emphasises choice, control and personal responsibility and fits in well with the personal/consumer perspective which stresses taking control of your own health. But it also has a more subtle political agenda: 'Don't blame us if you are ill, or expect us to pay for your health care. It's your fault; you should be looking after yourself.'

Stories and issues
A story may become a peg on which coverage of an issue can be hung, but real, human interest events are often needed if a topic is to get widespread coverage. An event may be covered as a story and then picked up as an issue for documentary or feature coverage. Sometimes too much focus on an event may obscure the issues. In healthcare reporting this can be counter-productive. Reports that don't give the supporting knowledge needed to give meaning to events often lead to fear, anger and indignation which healthcare professionals then have to deal with.

News media try to fit experience into established frameworks. Look at the two photographs of the Moors murderer Myra Hindley on page 25, then read the extract below.

'Myra Hindley looked nothing whatsoever like her famous photograph, the tarty-looking picture with the white-blonde hair and the big, bulging eyes, the evil Moors Murderess. She seemed timid, with a shy, little-girl-lost manner that I was reminded of, years later, by Princess Diana. Hindley really didn't look capable of the gruesome child killings that had sent her to prison.'

Jones, J. and Clerk, C. (1993) *The Devil and Miss Jones*. London: Smith Gryphon.

What is striking about the description?

EYES: Medium

HAIR: Medium

WEIGHT: Medium

HEIGHT: Medium

DISTINGUISHING FEATURES: None

NUMBER OF FINGERS: Ten

NUMBER OF TOES: Ten

INTELLIGENCE: Medium

What did you expect?

Talons?
Oversize incisors?
Green saliva?
Madness?

Leonard Cohen (1969) All there is to know about Adolph Eichmann. *Selected Poems 1956-1968*. London: Jonathan Cape.

Mediating experience

What people read, hear or see is not firsthand experience, and can never be the same as a firsthand experience. In mediating experiences, the media necessarily select, interpret and colour the experience. Reality is not mediated only once — the news we hear about is not something that happened to the reporter, but something that has been reported to the reporter. Layers of meaning are added to the experience or event as it is mediated. Some of this is deliberate and conscious, some a matter of convenience, or the result of the pressures of the news-gathering and reporting process.

As you study the media, you will become more aware of the codes that allow material to be presented in a digestible and familiar form. You can also look behind the codes to try to work out why the established norms are as they are. For example, Section 2 looks at some of the external influences on the way the media work and present information and interpretations.

Conspiracy theory

It may sometimes seem to you when you analyse media coverage of healthcare issues that there is a conspiracy to maintain the dominant modes of representation, to promote an agreed message and to uphold the establishment in its current form. Some media critics and specialists believe this to be the case (see pages 42–43). It is probably fairer, though, to see various economic and practical constraints at work. But the effect may be the same — the dominant ideology predominates, the voice of the establishment is given more scope than dissonant voices. Even so, people do not believe all they read, see or hear in the media; they apply common sense and a good dose of scepticism. And their interpretation of media reports often includes a critical assessment of accuracy and reliability compared to the touchstones of their own ideas and experiences.

Section 2 focuses on aspects of media influence which, when taken alone, may suggest a conspiracy between the ruling classes and the media to maintain the status quo. However, Section 4, which focuses on how the media impact on our lives and on society as a whole,

---

A quantitative study of the media coverage given to victims of violence and political injustice found that US media outlets gave considerably more space to victims of régimes seen to oppose the US dominant ideology than to victims of supposed 'friendly' powers. (Herman, E. and Chomsky, N. (1988) *Manufacturing Consent*. New York and Toronto: Random House.)

What are the possible reasons for this disparity in coverage? Do the reasons you identify suggest a 'conspiracy theory' reading of media activity or are there more practical reasons to account for the differences?

'...broadcasting can be diagnosed as a new and powerful form of social integration and control. Many of its main uses can be seen as socially, commercially and at times politically manipulative.'

Williams, R. (1990) *Television: Technology and cultural form*. London: Routledge (second edition).

'Television alone (or with other media) is not responsible for shaping a generation's way of thinking...If the generation goes against what television invited it to do (while showing signs of having fully absorbed its expressive forms and mental operations), it has read television differently from most of those who produce it, those who consume it and the sum total of the theoreticians analysing it.'

Eco, U. (1995) *Apocalypse Postponed*. London: HarperCollins.

draws on issues that would seem to contradict a conspiracy theory. The panel below suggests how to ask critical questions about the role of the media and come to your own conclusions. Some of your answers may put different interpretations on media activity; others may support the notion of a conspiracy.

The role and function of the media

The media exist partly to inform and entertain. But by taking a wider look at the social role of the media, it is possible to see other functions it may fulfil. As you study the media, think about what you feel their role should be. Should the media be in the control of the state to educate, to develop culture, to promote social unity? Should they be in the hands of the people, for socialisation, to develop popular culture, and encourage cultural diversity? To help you formulate your own views you may find it helpful to look at pages 40–41 which outline some of the ways in which media theorists have formulated the role of the media in society, and then read the panel below which suggests several ways of looking at the role of the media in different areas.

A critical attitude

A critical attitude to the media means recognising the variety of viewpoints and voices that abound, identifying their source and bias and analysing their significance. News and information is normally presented from one perspective; readers or viewers are drawn in and 'get the picture' from the perspective of the presenter. If they have a well-developed perspective of their own, they can resist the presenter's perspective and look at what is being reported from a different point of view. It is necessary to develop critical antennae towards the media. Because health issues are presented regularly throughout the media, healthcare professionals will benefit from developing their antennae and casting a critical eye on what they — and their patients — see, hear and read.

There are many ways of thinking about the media and how they influence our lives and our view of the world. The questions that arise suggest possible opposing interpretations of the role and function of the media.

Talk with colleagues about which interpretations are closest to your own and think about these issues. You will probably find that you have quite complex answers that include some apparently contradictory elements. Do you need to reconcile your ideas or are you happy to accommodate the contradictions?

The media and culture. Do the media:

- Maintain continuity and help us to define and understand our culture?
- Offer opportunities for sub-cultures to find expression and reach a larger audience?
- Reinforce the mass culture at the expense of cultural diversity?
- Maintain the status quo and discourage growth?

The media and society. Do the media:

- Provide a model of society that helps us to operate within society as it is?
- Provide a forum for discussion and a way for dissonant or marginal voices to be heard?
- Naturalise one view of society at the expense of alternative views?

The media and entertainment. Do the media:

- Provide pleasing entertainment to occupy people's leisure time?
- Distract people from real activity?
- Distract people from thinking about important social and political issues (an 'opiate of the people')?

The media and information. Do the media:

- Provide valuable information to help us live our lives and make decisions in an open and informed climate?
- Promote a particular view of the world by selecting and presenting information?

The media and politics. Do the media:

- Represent political events and processes so that we can understand and partake of them more fully?
- Endorse the established order?
- Mobilise public opinion following their own agenda or that of the established order?
- Offer opportunities for diversity and to challenge the established order?

Conclusion

This Section has raised many issues which are returned to in the rest of the book. They may be useful 'threads' for you to hang your thoughts on as you work through the book. Keep a look out for these threads:

- Tensions between the messages intended in a media report and the messages you receive
- The reader's or viewer's role in constructing the message
- Any hidden agendas in reports
- The dominant ideology behind the presentation of stories
- Codes of language and pictures that media presenters share with readers and viewers
- How stories and events are fitted to established frameworks
- How the media are influenced and how the media exert influence
- The role of the media in reflecting and shaping public opinion and perceptions.

References

Dixon, B. (1994) A rampant non-epidemic. *British Medical Journal* 308: 1576.

Entwhistle, V. and Hancock-Beaulieu, M. (1992) Health and medical coverage in the UK national press. *Public Understanding of Science* 1(4): 367–82.

Hartley, J. (1982) *Understanding News*. London: Methuen. (Reprinted 1988, Routledge, London.)

Herman, E. and Chomsky, N. (1988) *Manufacturing Consent*. New York and Toronto: Random House.

Karpf, A. (1988) *Doctoring the Media. The reporting of health and medicine*. London: Routledge.

McLuhan, M. (1964) *Understanding Media: The extensions of man*. London: Routledge (reprinted 1994).

Parkin, F. In: Hartley, J. (1982). *Understanding News*. London: Methuen. (Reprinted 1988, Routledge.)

Smith, J. (1996) The value of nursing journals. (Editorial.) *Journal of Advanced Nursing* 24(1): 1–2.

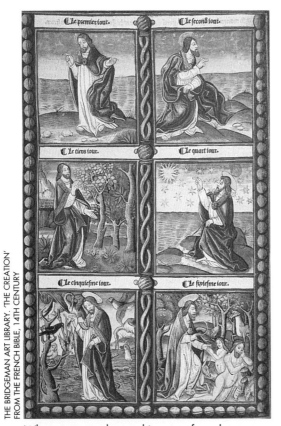

THE BRIDGEMAN ART LIBRARY. 'THE CREATION' FROM THE FRENCH BIBLE, 14TH CENTURY

What can you select and interpret from these images?

Make notes for yourself in your learning journal about any questions that have been raised in this Section.

Do you have answers to any of the questions?

Do you feel you need to think more deeply, or look at more evidence?

Are there aspects of investigating the media where you don't yet know what you think?

Are there questions not raised in this Section that you think are important?

You may like to write a critique of this Section and how well it has handled the issues raised, or discuss the questions above with others in your tutor/counsellor group.

Introduction

This Section looks at the day-to-day operation of news-gathering and production. It also investigates the complex interplay of influences, controls and regulations that determine what gets into the media, including:

- External influences on what is published or broadcast, such as the state, economic constraints, public relations
- Legal restrictions and statutory obligations which affect what is published or broadcast
- Internal constraints within the media, such as production processes.

It is useful to know about these things for two reasons. Understanding the internal and external pressures on reporters, editors and programme-makers helps to explain:

- How and why they take the decisions they do about the content and presentation of stories
- The subtle, shifting relationships between different versions of events — for example, what the government says about an industrial dispute and what the union says.

You will be looking at items that have made it into the media — because you can't look at what is not there. But some stories never get into the press or onto the airwaves. They may be subject to censorship, suppression or cannot be published because of statutory or regulatory restrictions. Other stories break at the wrong time, are displaced by something more dramatic or are regarded as being too dull to be covered, even if they are important.

There are several models of how the media work within society to influence and reflect opinion. Two are shown in the diagram below. This Section will encourage you to think about how you believe the media are acted upon in relation to these and other models. It looks briefly at advertising in the media, but considers fiction only in the context of television — the one medium in which fact and fiction are constantly found side by side.

Flora Keays is the daughter of Sara Keays and ex-Conservative party chairman Sir Cecil Parkinson. She has suffered numerous health problems, but her mother has been unable to campaign in the press for the special help her daughter needs because of a gagging order, which prevents photographs of Flora being published.

'Sara Keays believes that publicity might enable her to campaign successfully for better educational treatment for her daughter, in particularly campaigning with her local authority to meet Flora's special needs'. Bevins, A., Price., J. (1996) Exposed: the court gag that has silenced Sara Keays. *Observer*, January 28, 1996, page 1.

'Injunctions were imposed against Sara Keays to protect Cecil Parkinson and not to protect their daughter's interests, sources close to the litigation claim.' Bevins, A., London; Bhatia, S., Jerusalem. (1996) Keays gagged 'to shield Parkinson'. *Observer*, February 4, 1996, page 1.

A critical attitude to the media means not always accepting their version of the facts as truthful and authentic. What would make you think that these *Observer* reports are either biased or relatively unbiased?

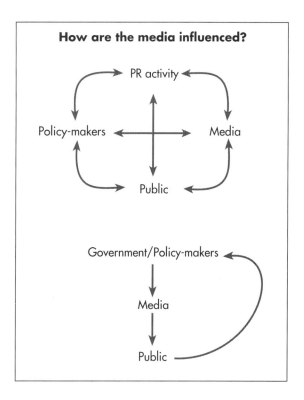

How are the media influenced?

Models of mass communication

Media theories attempt to define the way the media work — how they relate to society and the state, how they communicate with people and the part they play in social and political processes. Two opposing poles in media theory are dominance and pluralism:

- *Dominance:* sees the media controlled by and in the service of a dominant class or élite group
- *Pluralism:* sees a range of media fragmented by disparate beliefs, attitudes and directions and responding to demand from the public (Abercrombie, 1980).

A dominant media theorist would see the quashing of the *Cook Report's* investigation into sudden infant death syndrome (The Cot-death Poisonings', Central TV, November 17 and December 1, 1994) as evidence of the establishment discrediting a threatening theory. A pluralist interpretation would see the diversity of reporting on the issue, from the *Cook Report's* own programme to the varied follow-up on television and in other media, as evidence of the many voices and interests represented by the media.

The diagram below locates schools of media theory on the line between dominance and pluralism. The rest of these two pages summarise the main thinking behind some of these theories.

Marxist theories are based on the premise that organisations are controlled by and serve the current power-holders. Contemporary Marxists argue that the media disseminate the ideas of the ruling class and deny alternative ideas which might empower the working classes. The first three categories below are Marxist theories.

Political-economic theory

This suggests that the economics of the market and media ownership are a more important influence than ideology. 'Uneconomic' sectors of the market are ignored or under-represented, there is a move towards large conglomerates and away from independent media sources, risk-taking in reporting is reduced and those who have a voice are those least likely to challenge the status quo.

Critical theory

According to the Frankfurt school of thought, individuals and society are dependent on the picture of the world presented to them through the media to define their thinking. As a result, capitalism has been 'sold' to the masses and

Main dimensions and locations of media theory

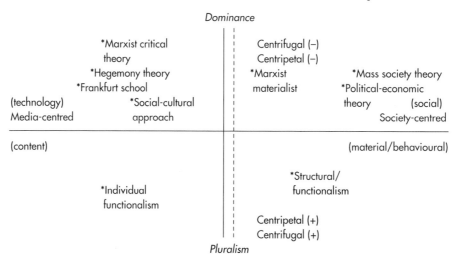

Source: McQuail, D. (1987) *Mass Communication Theory. An introduction.* London: Sage Publications (second edition), p59.

become the dominant social force; social change is prevented and natural social growth and diversity stifled.

Media hegemony

Ideology is central to this interpretation. The media are seen as 'a pervasive and deliberate cultural influence which serve to interpret experience of reality in a covert but consistent manner' (McQuail, 1987). Politicians, proprietors and other powerful groups in society use the media to encourage people to accept and assimilate the dominant ideology.

Mass society theory

This stresses the integration of the media into the sources of power and authority in society. The content of the media serves the interests of those who already hold power, and endorses a view of the world as it already is, helping people to locate and understand their place in it. It both helps maintain the current *status quo* and helps people deal with their lot.

Culturalist or social-cultural approach

This looks at the meaning of popular culture and how various groups in society respond to it. The aim is to see how mass culture helps to integrate and subordinate potentially deviant or oppositional elements. Instead of the media reflecting society, it sees mass culture as integrated with all social activity: people make choices about media consumption and about the messages they take and use on the basis of their experience within social groups.

Functionalist approaches

This sees the activities of society as responses to its needs. The function of the media is to give a reasonably accurate picture of society and to respond to the needs of individuals and groups within society. 'Structural-functional theory. . . depicts media as essentially self-directing and self-correcting, within certain politically negotiated institutional rules' (McQuail, 1987). Post-modernist theories fit into this approach. They suggest that people make their own representations of experience, including experience of the media, using them to form a self-image and a lifestyle. There is a complex and sophisticated layer of 'transaction' between the media and how they are received — people are to some extent in control of these transactions, although the media itself may convey powerful suggestions of images and lifestyles (Giddens, 1986).

This Section of the book focuses on issues and ideas that may tend to support dominance theories. Section 4 focuses on issues and concerns that tend to support pluralist theories. As you work on the Activities in both Sections, keep all the models in mind and come to your own conclusions about the relative merits of different theories. You could also try to position the model you favour in relation to dominance and pluralism.

If you want to find out more about media theory and mass communications, read:

McQuail, D. (1987) *Mass Communication Theory: An introduction*. London: Sage Publications (second edition).

You might want to investigate critically some of these theories as part of your assessment for this unit. For example, you could apply a range of theories to one or more events and use them to account for the ways these events were represented in the media.

Alternatively, you might like to explore how particular models of the role and function of the media in society enable people to think differently about the 'transactional' relationship between the media and their audiences.

Make notes in your learning journal on how you need to review or accommodate ideas differently according to the model(s) of the media you choose to use.

The state and the media

In a democracy, citizens expect open government and a say in policy decisions. They may not always get it. Many overt and covert influences are at work. One way in which the state can manipulate people's perception of what is happening and what are the significant issues is by trying to manage or control media reporting. The box below gives an example about the leaked findings of a government inquiry into diet and how the government tried to bias the findings and suppress the report.

A heritage of political influence

The impact of the state on the media is far-reaching. The government is in a particularly privileged position as it can, if necessary, legislate to get its own way. It also has the ability to release and withhold information as it sees fit, to further its own ends. In the 18th and 19th centuries, the approved newspapers were commonly financed and provided with information by the government. The last paper to receive a government subsidy was the *Observer*, which gave it up in 1845 in favour of increased independence. But the government still controls the flow of information, through channels such as:

- Official statements, press conferences and press releases (see pages 114–117)
- Briefings in which government spokespeople talk to journalists directly
- Government press offices making available previously-released reports.

When the BBC began public service broadcasting in 1927, its Director General, John Reith, was keen to avoid political intervention. The government, on its part, was keen to avoid being embroiled in what it considered to be a trivial affair, so the BBC was left largely to its own devices. This was to change. Broadcasts were closely monitored during the Second World War for reasons of national security, but state intervention extended beyond the end of the war. Criticism that the BBC shows bias came from governments of all political persuasions, and continues to this day. Sometimes the criticism takes a more official tone which may result in direct intervention, such as the withdrawal of a *Real Lives* broadcast in 1985 because the government did not want the IRA to have a voice on national television. Independent television and the press are less obviously subject to government regulation because they are not state institutions. The influencing process is not fail-safe — the

'Mounting poverty during 16 years of Conservative rule has produced malnutrition among Britons on a scale unseen since the 1930s. An unpublished government report leaked to the *Observer* concludes that urgent action needs to be taken to improve the diet of millions of Britains. The report is deeply embarrassing to the Government and the inquiry team was forbidden from discussing or recommending what some of its members believe to be an essential prerequisite to healthier eating — the raising of state benefits. Opposition and consumer groups will seize upon the report as a damning indictment of the Government's welfare and economic policies.'

Jones, J.(1996) Poverty triggers UK diet crisis. *Observer*, January 21, 1996.

'There is a widespread belief in political circles — although this is not necessarily shared by the general public — that news and current affairs on television are neither objective nor impartial and that they are, in fact, persistently biased in favour of the Left.'

Introduction to the first report of the Media Monitoring Unit, written by Lord Chalfont. Quoted in: Philo, G. (ed) (1995) Television, politics and the rise of the new right. *Glasgow Media Group Reader. Volume 2.* London: Routledge.

media often resist the pressures put on them and have their own sources of information. For example, they can get information about what happens in government by direct media presence at Westminster. They can also look up the exact words used in a debate in the full daily proceedings published by the Hansard Society. These are the official channels, which give direct access to open proceedings. But they do not give access to closed sessions, the meetings of committees and private Cabinet discussions. These are reported, selectively, in documents and statements issued by the government. Sometimes committee reports may be suppressed or their publication played down if they are unfavourable to the government. Another tactic is to release a more important or topical piece of news, to take attention away from the publication of an unfavourable report.

There are also unofficial sources, including whistle-blowers and leaks. Some leaks have official sanction. These are the result of a government department deciding that information should be available to the public but should not be released in the government's own voice. Government sources may sometimes also engineer leaks as a damage limitation exercise.

Politics and the media

Philo (1995) has identified three key issues in the relationship between politics and the media since the start of the 1980s:

- A sustained attack by the government on news and current affairs broadcasting, especially on the BBC, including the setting up of the Media Monitoring Unit headed by the right-wing politician Lord Chalfont (later appointed as deputy chairman of the Independent Television Commission — formerly the Independent Broadcasting Authority (IBA)
- Extensive use of the media and public relations to promote political ideology
- New legislative structures which constrain broadcasters and attack the 'public service' ethos of the BBC; for example, the new Official Secrets Act 1989 preventing civil servants from making 'damaging disclosures' to the press, and the Broadcasting Act 1990 extending deregulation of radio and TV.

Labour as well as Conservative governments have complained of bias in the BBC's reporting. Is this most likely to indicate that:

- There is no significant bias?
- The bias changes with time, for example, over the lifetime of a government?

An interesting article investigating allegations of bias is: Miller, D. (1993) The Beeb at bay. *British Journalism Review* 4 (1): 20-26.

Mrs Thatcher's press secretary, Bernard Ingham, held weekly meetings with all the heads of information from the main government departments. A 'senior Whitehall figure' told the political journalist Robert Harris that the purpose of these meetings was 'ensuring bits of good news don't clash, masking bad news at one department by bringing forward good from another...deciding whether a television producer, on past experience, is to be trusted and so on'.

Harris, R. (1983) *Gotcha! The Media, the Government and the Falklands Crisis.* London: Faber.

'Questions asked by backbench members of Parliament [on the use of NHS money and prioritisation] produce all too frequently the reply that this information is not held centrally. It could be argued that this is a form of censorship imposed by government.'

Neuberger, J. (1994) What sort of information should be available to the public in an open society? In: Marinker, M. (ed) (1994) *Controversies in Health Care Policies: Challenges to practice.* London: BMA Publishing.

Is it fair to say that the way information is collected and held may be a form of censorship?

What examples do you know of in health care where information is not made freely available, either to the media or to other researchers?

Regulation and control

What gets into the papers and on to television and radio is chosen on a day-to-day basis by editors and producers. They determine an editorial policy that ensures consistency and follows the agenda of the broadcaster or publisher. But who sets the agenda? A combination of internal and external influences affect both the agenda and the final content.

Whatever a publisher or broadcaster wants to produce is also subject to regulation and limitation by various codes, bodies and statutes. These make the media accountable to external bodies for their activities. There are both statutory and voluntary codes which attempt to regulate what gets into the media. The regulatory framework has several aims:
- Maintaining political balance
- Protecting the state
- Protecting individuals
- Providing material that is 'good' for people
- Providing opportunities for different sectors of the community to be heard.

Regulations for different media

There are regulatory bodies for different forms of the media and laws relating both to specific media and to the media in general.

The laws relevant to media output are:
- Broadcasting Act 1990, governing radio and television
- Obscene Publications Act 1959, governing press and cinema but not broadcasting; it aims to protect people from material 'likely to corrupt or deprave'
- Defamation laws on libel and slander, which apply to all forms of the media
- Contempt of Court Act 1981, preventing the media reporting on anything that may affect the outcome of a case that is *sub judice*
- Official Secrets Act 1989, preventing the media publishing or broadcasting anything that might be considered against the 'national interest'.

As well as these laws, the activities of the BBC are dictated by its Licence and Agreement and the activities of independent television are regulated by the ITC (and previously by the IBA). The BBC is bound by its charter to observe due balance and impartiality in its programming. It also has to provide a range of programming to cater to different tastes. Some of the programmes must be educational. The ITC also requires independent television channels to observe balance and impartiality

The Independent Broadcasting Authority (IBA) charter states that it shall be the duty of the Authority to ensure that:

- Programmes broadcast maintain a proper balance and wide range in their subject matter

- All news given in the programmes (in whatever form) is presented with due accuracy and impartiality

- Due impartiality is preserved on the part of the persons providing the programmes as respects matters of political or industrial controversy or relating to current political policy.

IBA Charter. In: *Health, the Mass Media and the National Health Service*. London: Unit for the Study of Health Policy, Department of Community Medicine, Guy's Hospital Medical School, p63.

'Do You Wish to Vote for the Leaders of Law, Order, Peace and Prosperity? Or to Vote for the Overthrow of Society and Pave the Way to Bolshevism?'

Daily Mirror, October 29, 1924.

The proprietor of another daily newspaper, the *Daily Express*, told the Royal Commission on the Press that he ran the *Daily Express* 'merely for the purpose of making propaganda, and with no other motive'.

Quoted by Curran, J. and Seaton, J. (1991) *Power Without Responsibility: The press and broadcasting in Britain* London: Routledge (fourth edition).

clauses and to provide a range of programming. If a channel does not follow the regulations, it risks losing its franchise. Channel 4 has a special remit to provide programming for special and minority interests. It is allowed to spread balance over its whole schedule, so it can present one point of view very strongly in a single programme as long as an opposing view is given air-time in some other programme. The activities of cable television are overseen (not regulated) by the Cable Authority.

There are four voluntary bodies that act as watchdogs over the media:
- Press Complaints Commission (established 1991): adjudicates complaints against the press; although it has no power to enforce its judgements, papers tend to comply.
- Advertising Standards Authority (established 1962): aims to ensure that all advertisements are 'legal, decent, honest and truthful'; it has the support of the advertising industry but no legal powers of enforcement
- Broadcasting Standards Council (established under the Broadcasting Act in 1990, but existing 'in shadow' since 1988): monitors the portrayal of sex and violence and matters of taste and decency, examines complaints and publishes its findings in a monthly bulletin; though independent and advisory, it exerts pressure on the industry
- Broadcasting Complaints Commission (established 1981): handles complaints about intrusion of privacy and unjust treatment by broadcasting organisations.

Regulation and press freedom

Regulation is not intended to be censorship, but there are points at which it is reasonable to ask whether press freedom is being compromised. The balance between freedom of the press and protection of the public is a difficult one, and everyone interprets it slightly differently. Contentious cases in recent years include:
- The *Sunday Times* was found in contempt of court during the thalidomide hearings when it put the interests of the victims above the restrictions on reporting the trial
- Civil servant Sarah Tisdall was jailed for releasing Ministry of Defence information to the *Guardian*, contravening the Official Secrets Act.

'We define the freedom of the press as that freedom from restraint which is essential to enable proprietors, editors and journalists to advance the public interest by publishing the facts and opinions without which a democratic electorate cannot make responsible judgements.'

Royal Commission on the Press (1974-1977). *Final Report* (1977). London: HMSO, Cmnd 6810.

How could the above definition of press freedom be extended or improved? For example, what are the limits on how proprietors, editors and journalists should exercise their freedom? What protection is there against abuse of freedom, such as the invasion of personal limits or the distortion of remarks made in good faith?

Pressure groups and lobbying

How do politicians decide which policies to pursue or how to vote in a debate? How do decision-makers gather information on which to base decisions? And how can interests in the community be furthered? Politicians receive a lot of information — some which they ask for and some which they don't — from pressure groups representing different views and factions. The process by which a group tries to influence government is called lobbying. A pressure group may represent any group of people or interest, from a commercial group (such as the British Poultry Meat Federation) to an environmental cause (such as Friends of the Earth).

Types of pressure groups

There is a huge number of pressure groups in the UK — probably tens of thousands. Political writers divide them into three main types:

- *Primary and secondary pressure groups*
  Primary pressure groups are those whose main aim is political influence. Secondary pressure groups are those whose main aim is something other than political influence, but who become involved in political action and lobbying to further their aims
- *'Cause' and sectional groups.* A 'cause' group represents a belief or principle and acts to

further its cause. A sectional group represents a particular section of society. Generally, cause groups have a larger membership and wider aims; sectional groups concentrate on restricted issues with narrower appeal to the public and often have more resources with which to pursue their aims
- *'Insider' and 'outsider' groups.* An insider group is one regarded as legitimate by the government and regularly consulted by it. An outsider group is one which does not want or cannot gain close alliance with the government. Generally, insider groups have a better chance of influencing policy decisions. They 'play by the rules', use accepted political tactics and skills, and use the same language as senior civil servants and ministers.

How pressure groups work

Pressure groups try to achieve their aims by several strategies, including:

- Negotiation with government — setting up meetings with ministers
- Persuading individual politicians to vote for or against a particular motion, perhaps using petitions and mail-shots
- Media exposure to make the public more aware and concerned about an issue or group

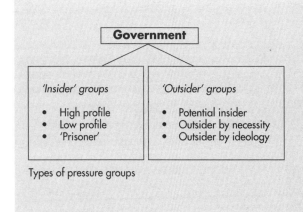

Types of pressure groups

'An important point about the insider/outsider distinction is that it highlights the way in which the state sets the rules of the game for pressure group activity. Access and consultation flow from the adoption of a pattern of behaviour which is acceptable to government, particularly to civil servants. This creates incentives for groups to act in a particular way; pressure groups are thus tamed and domesticated with only the ideological rejectionists remaining outside the system.'

Grant, W. (1995) *Pressure Groups, Politics and Democracy in Britain.* Hemel Hempstead: Philip Allan (second edition).

- Official consultation by invitation with government officials, departments, committees and ministers
- Direct action, such as sabotaging fox-hunts.

Many pressure groups use the media extensively to try to get their case heard and to further their aims. They may:
- Arrange events and release reports which bring their group into the news temporarily
- Initiate documentaries and features about their work or their cause
- Advertise directly — large groups such as Amnesty International and Friends of the Earth have a substantial advertising budget; they issue press releases and hold press conferences to keep their case in the public eye and keep the media informed.

Pressure groups often polarise around producers and consumers. In general, the producers have more focused goals and form a more cohesive group. They are likely to be better resourced and more sophisticated. Consumer groups often have more disparate interests and membership profiles. So a group of consultants trying to get a change in hospital policy stand more chance of success than a group of patients. The patients

are likely to be motivated by different personal interests and experiences. Although their feelings may be strong, they will not all share the same interests and experiences. There will be more uniformity in the aims and experiences of the consultants. The media tend to support consumer groups; this gives the groups increased exposure and impact which helps to balance the better resourcing and organisation of producer groups.

Relationships between media and the state suggest that political parties are sometimes anxious about media bias and concerned to regulate their activities. Since anxiety comes from across the political spectrum, this does not at first suggest that the media hold a uniform ideological position. But what truth is there in the claim that they represent a relatively narrow range of views and tend to exclude alternative views? (Illich, 1972.)

Is the existence of pressure groups beneficial or detrimental to the democratic process? If you know of a case where a pressure group has influenced decisions about health care, you might like to investigate it as part of your assessment for the unit. Or you could discuss the question in general terms with others in your tutor/counsellor group.

'A pressure group is an organisation which seeks as one of its functions to influence the formulation and implementation of public policy, said public policy representing a set of authoritative decisions taken by the executive, the legislature, and the judiciary, and by local government and the European Union.'

Grant W. (1995) *Pressure Groups, Politics and Democracy in Britain*. Hemel Hempstead: Philip Allan (second edition).

For an interesting account of how a pressure group with a very particular aim maintained press interest, read the account of the attempts by the Friends of John McCarthy to secure his release from Beirut and of those who were taken hostage with him in :

Morrell, J. and McCarthy, J. (1993) *Some Other Rainbow*. London: Bantam Press.

In a debate about reducing or raising the latest point in pregnancy when an abortion may be performed, politicians may be lobbied by church and other religious groups and groups with moral concerns, medical and healthcare professionals, pro-life groups and pro-choice groups. The government may seek advice from medical ethics philosophers.

How is your profession represented in the lobbying and pressure group system? How has this representation influenced:
- The way the profession is viewed and respected by the government?
- Legislation directly or indirectly related to the profession?

Economic influences

The economic influences and constraints on the media are considerable. They affect:
- Who can own a newspaper or broadcast organisation
- Who is represented by the media
- Whose interests are served by the media
- Which subjects are covered
- The form in which topics are covered
- The presentation and order of materials.

A brief history of media economics

Two hundred years ago, almost anyone could start a paper: a radical press emerged alongside the burgeoning trade unions and radical political movement (Thompson, 1968). The start-up cost was low, and a paper could survive on its cover price alone — it was self-financing just from its circulation. The only requirement of the editorial content was to appeal to sufficient literate people for the paper to pay its way. From the mid 19th century, printing technology became more advanced and the cost of production rose. As a result, the radical press declined, and the political spectrum represented by published newspapers grew narrower. Only richer people were able to start up a paper, and so papers produced by and for the working classes declined.

As the cost of producing a paper increased, publishers could not raise the cover price of their papers sufficiently to cover costs and had to find other methods of financing them. These days the cover price of a newspaper no longer covers even the cost of the paper and ink, and certainly does not pay for its production and distribution, although some specialist newsletters can survive on circulation alone. Advertising has emerged as the main source of revenue, as it has for independent television companies.

The impact of advertising

Advertisers have commercial goals. They will advertise in a publication or on a broadcast channel only if the advertising leads to enough sales to cover costs and generate extra profit. For advertisers in newspapers, this means that sales of the paper must be:
- Big enough to reach a sufficient market for the product
- To readers with enough money to buy the goods
- To readers who want to buy the goods.

On television, the audience has a wider spread of social profile. Advertisers aim at reaching as many people as possible in the hope that they will catch

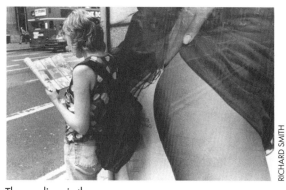

The medium is the message

Here the Word has withered to a few
Parched certainties, and the charred stubble
Tightens like a black belt, a crop of Bibles...

These are the places where the Spirit dies.
And now, in Desertmartin's sandy light,
I see a culture of twigs and bird-shit
Waving a gaudy flag it loves and curses.
Tom Paulin (1983) Desertmartin. In: *Liberty Tree*.
London: Faber and Faber.

the viewers they want — their target market. They will take opportunities to reach a more carefully targeted audience when these arise, but this cannot be their usual method of operation. Changes in broadcasting patterns towards 'narrowcasting' — programming targeted at smaller and more carefully defined groups — mean that this is likely to change in the near future.

Advertising inevitably affects editorial policy. Publications and broadcast channels may not be able to give prominence to reports or features that will alienate the advertisers on which they depend. If the readership drops off or changes profile, the advertisers will go elsewhere. The balance works the other way as well: readership may drop off if the editor kow-tows to the advertisers too obviously, so that the editorial loses its 'bite'. The editorial board has to achieve and maintain a delicate balance if the publication is to survive.

Besides readers of the right type, a publication needs the right number of readers. (The same is true to a lesser extent of the audiences of broadcast media.) A paper or magazine needs either many readers with a little money, or a few

readers with a lot of money. A broadsheet needs a smaller circulation to survive than does a tabloid. Again, there must be a balance. The left-wing *Daily Herald* closed in 1965, even though it had a circulation of one-and-a-half million, because its circulation was not large enough to support the type of advertising it depended upon. On the other hand, the *Times* suffered a crisis when it increased its circulation and lost advertisers. The reader profile changed — moving downmarket — as the cover price dropped and the circulation increased.

Collect three or four different types of publication, for example, a broadsheet and tabloid newspaper, a women's weekly magazine, a professional health-related journal. Look at the type of advertising each carries for healthcare products and services.

What can you tell about the readership each is aiming at from the advertising it carries?

How do you think maintaining these advertisers affects the editorial policy of the publication? Look through the editorial to see whether you can find evidence to support your expectations.

Pressure from readers led some women's magazines to drop advertisements for cigarettes in the 1980s. Fears of reduced circulation because readers opposed advertising for an unhealthy product became more financially compelling than the desire for revenue from the cigarette manufacturers.

On the day Microsoft released its Windows 95 operating system for PCs, it subsidised every copy of the *Times* so that the paper was free. Besides promoting Microsoft's product, this would distort the circulation figures for the Times making it look more attractive to other advertisers.

On January 21, 1996, Waterstone's book shops joined up with the *Observer* in a promotional campaign. The paper was given away free in Waterstone's shops. Every free copy of the *Observer* was counted in the circulation figures and so distorted the circulation figures that would be issued by the Audit Bureau of Circulation (ABC).

Do we get what we want or want what we get?

Market theory suggests that market forces operate to make available the products which people want to buy: the balance of media available should represent what people want to read, listen to and watch. This is not necessarily the case. About 13 million national daily newspapers are sold each day. Many will be read by more than one person in a household. There are perhaps 25 million or so readers. But this does not mean that most of the adult population can read the paper they want. They can only choose from those that are presented to them.

Combined influences

Section 3 looks in more detail at influences on the content and ownership of the media. Many of these influences work together to determine the forms of the media available:

- The content and balance of programmes on the BBC is restricted to some extent by its charter, and influenced by the need to keep viewers in order to justify the licence fee
- Independent television and radio channels have to balance satisfying advertisers (by attracting viewers) and satisfying the ITC (by observing its guidelines) in order to keep their franchises

- Advertising determines the market for a newspaper and influences its content
- A publication needs a balance of advertising and circulation to pay its way; a publication aimed at people with low incomes may not be viable
- The allocation of resources affects which news can be covered and which programmes made
- Established notions of newsworthiness and the practical constraints of the news-gathering process determine which items get into the news, though these may not be the items that people would be most interested in
- The possibilities of foreign sales and syndication make broadcasters aware of the requirements of the global market, perhaps at the expense of the tastes and preferences of the home market.

Success and failure

One way of analysing the commercial requirements of a channel or publication is to look at those that have failed and find out why they did not work. Presumably they answered some consumer demand or they would never have existed. It clearly was not adequate to counter other factors or they would not have failed.

'It is occasionally indicated to us that we are apparently setting out to give the public what we think they need and not what they want — but few know what they want, and very few what they need.'

Lord Reith, Director General of the BBC, quoted In: Curran, J. and Seaton, J. (1991) *Power Without Responsibility: The press and broadcasting in Britain*. London: Routledge (fourth edition, p139).

'In a free market economy, consumers can only buy that which is offered to them, and that which is offered is not necessarily that which is most advantageous. It is that which appears to give the prospect of profit to the producer.'

Lord Beveridge. Ibid; p135. [A remark made in 1934.]

What would you like to see in a magazine, newspaper or television channel? If you had the chance to propose a new addition to a publication or broadcast programme, what would you propose? Think about the issues that would affect it:

Would it attract advertising?

Would enough people be interested in it?

Why do you think it doesn't exist already?

'Art is giving way to the postures of Culture and the wrapping of Reichstags. The art of living is arbitrated in consumer troughs called supermarkets. Reflection is replaced by the global inanities of a CNN cancelling out values and destroying the capacity for memory and discernment and citizen participation.'

Breytenbach, B. (1996) *The Memory of Birds in Times of Revolution*. Cape Town: Human & Rousseau.

The success or failure of a media outlet is not necessarily an indication of its popularity with the public but depends largely on various market forces. Here are some examples:

- The *Today* newspaper was closed by Rupert Murdoch in spite of bids to buy it out, partly because it competed with his other interests
- The satellite channel BSB was taken over by Sky and disappeared after initial talks of a merger
- *Marxism Today* closed after the dissolution of the Communist party
- The feminist magazine *Spare Rib* closed as a result of the changing socio-political climate
- The *Listener* magazine was closed down by the BBC following falling circulation
- The *Sunday Correspondent* closed because there was too much competition in its market niche; it lost advertisers to the newly launched *Independent on Sunday*.

How they persuade 'us'

Newspapers persuade readers that they are providing what they want by creating an identity as one of 'us'. The 'us' they represent is as wide-ranging as possible to include the largest possible market. Tabloid papers might feed on and create an appetite for popular prejudices and preconceptions about subjects such as law and order, concern for good health care and education, and patriotism in foreign affairs, particularly wars. In the 1980s, the *Sun* became notorious for adopting a populist stance that reflected public feeling — supporting the death penalty, for instance. The 'quality' papers have a different view of 'us'. Again 'we' support law and order and Britain, though maybe more thoughtfully so. But 'we' are also interested in business, finance, justice and other 'serious' matters.

This created identity and empathy generate a 'feel good factor' which persuades readers that the paper is giving us what we want. It might also be capable of changing 'our' desires and views in accordance with its own.

''Why do you English have so many papers?' It was difficult to come up with a simple answer. Habit? Because we are such a tolerant and plural democracy? I think the main reason is because journalists like working for them. There is certainly no indication that the public demands them.'

Faulks, S. (1996) Ink-carnate. *Guardian*, March 5, 1996.

'To give the public what it wants is a misleading phrase... it has the appearance of an appeal to democratic principle, but the appearance is deceptive. It is in fact patronising and arrogant, in that it claims to know what the public is but defines it as no more than the mass audience, and it claims to know what it wants, but limits its choice to the average of experience.'

The Commission on Broadcasting. *Report presented to the Right Honourable John Reginald Bevins, PC, MP, Her Majesty's Postmaster General, on 5th June, 1962. (The Pilkington Report.)* London: HMSO, Cmnd 1753.

Reader/viewer response forums give audiences the chance to write in with their views and criticisms of coverage. They give the impression that the media are accountable and responsive to consumers. But how do the media respond? What evidence is there that people's opinions have an effect on editors or programme-makers?

Media 'surrounds'

Information is all around us and the human mind is extraordinarily efficient at dealing with it. Most information is discounted or processed automatically, as in the computational power needed to drive a car safely. Some information is noticed, for a variety of different reasons; for example, if, when we are driving, the lorry in front starts to veer into the middle of the road. Cognitive processes both ignore and take account of the surrounding data. The parallel processing, 'multitracking' ability of the mind allows us to receive, select and interpret multiple streams of data simultaneously (Dennett, 1991). To a great extent we are in control of what we receive.

McLuhan (1964) argued that in this century, we have 'extended our senses and our nerves by the various media'. This extension of ourselves by the use of television and electronic media has led to an 'implosion' of social and political functions and 'the substitution of the inclusive image for the mere viewpoint'. Because of their fragmentation and immediacy, the media (especially electronic media) have the power to convey multiple viewpoints; they have been instrumental in the shift from looking at things in sequence to looking at them in parallel —

what McLuhan calls the 'transition from lineal connections to configurations'. This simultaneous availability of information in different processed forms is what he meant by his famous phrase 'the medium is the message'.

Structuralists, such as the philosopher Roland Barthes, describe how a stream of information turns into signs that people can read like a sort of shorthand, without needing to look at every item. In his discussion of newspaper photographs, Roland Barthes draws attention to the 'complex of concurrent messages, with the photograph as centre and surrounds constituted by the text, the title, the caption, the layout and, in a more abstract but no less "informative" way, by the very name of the paper (this name represents a knowledge that can heavily orientate the reading of the message' (Barthes, 1983).

The concept of 'surrounds' introduced by Barthes is a useful one in relation to the media: it reminds us that the focus of attention is always influenced by what is around, in a wide sense of that word. Raymond Williams has documented the association of different forms of representation within the closed dimension of

---

'Cubism, by siezing on instant total awareness, suddenly announced that *the medium is the message*. Is it not evident that the moment that sequence yields to the simultaneous, one is in the world of the structure and of configuration? Is that not what has happened in physics as in painting, poetry and in communication? Specialized segments of attention have shifted to total field, and we can now say "The medium is the message" quite naturally.'

McLuhan, M. (1964) *Understanding Media: The extensions of man*. London: Routledge.

'The physical fact of instant transmission, as a technical possibility, has been uncritically raised to a social fact, without any pause to notice that virtually all such transmission is at once selected and controlled by existing social authorities. McLuhan, of course, would apparently do away with all such controls...'

Williams, R. (1990) *Television: Technology and cultural form*. London: Routledge.

'A tree is a tree. Yes, of course. But a tree as expressed by Minou Drouet is no longer quite a tree, it is a tree which is decorated, adapted to a certain type of consumption, laden with literary self-indulgence, revolt, images, in short with a type of social usage which is added to pure matter.'

Barthes, R. (1993). Myth today. In: Sontag, S. (ed) *A Roland Barthes Reader*. London: Vintage.

media (specifically television) programming, characterising it as a 'flow', which he relates directly to 'the growth and development of greater physical and social mobility' (Williams, 1975). Broadcasters may deal in timed units of 30 or 40 minutes but the experience of watching television breaks down this unitary perspective in two ways:

- There is considerable overspill and feedback from one unit to another, and within units — cumulatively, this effect of flow constitutes a powerful cultural message
- Memory, experience and attitudes are brought from outside, helping to break down or 'digest' the contents of a single unit or an evening's viewing. McLuhan (1964) described this as the breaking down of old, pre-electronic boundaries of space and time.

In his 'Perugia project', Umberto Eco took the analysis of the effects of television messages on viewers a stage further. This project identified some of the disjunctions between sender and receiver, which Eco describes in terms of codes and subcodes which may be more or less shared but which leave plenty of room for ambiguity, misunderstanding and interpretation. One of his conclusions was that 'television and radio news speak but the audience doesn't understand what they are saying' (Eco, 1995). He also started to categorise much wider types of viewer response, including responses such as day-dreaming and self-exclusion.

These considerations of the complexities surrounding the way media are received have profound implications for the relationship between sender and receiver. Far from being a pliant, receptive relationship, Eco characterises it as 'a semiological guerilla-warfare' in which interpretations clash and the interpretative process itself is constantly extended in a kind of decoding free-for-all.

World is suddener than we fancy it.

World is crazier and more of it than we think,
Incorrigibly plural. I peel and portion
A tangerine and spit the pips and feel
The drunkenness of things being various.
Louis MacNeice (1968) Snow. In: Hunter, J. (ed) *Modern Poets Three*. London: Faber.

The writers quoted on these pages disagree a lot with each other. But they all argue — in different ways — that media reporting gains significance less from the content of programmes or articles than from the resonances they set up with what people already know, think or feel. How true is this of your own experience of the media? As a 'receiver' of media messages, to what extent are you engaged in a 'guerilla-warfare' of interpretation and decoding?

Where do stories come from?

How does a story get into the news, or become the focus of a documentary or feature article? A lot is happening out there in the world but not all the interesting developments make it into the media. How do stories come to the attention of the reporters who might cover them?

Sources of news and features

The media feed off each other. An article that first appears in a local paper or on local radio may be picked up by the national papers and by national television and radio. A television story may be picked up by the newspapers. A development or discovery reported in the professional journals may be followed up in the papers and on television and radio. For healthcare stories, the professional journals and official reports are also important sources.

This explains how a story spreads, but not where it comes from. News is originally 'found' in one of four main ways:

- A press release is sent to papers and broadcasting organisations (about two-fifths of news stories are initiated by press departments)
- Reporters employed by a paper or broadcasting agency search out stories and keep in regular contact with the police and other likely sources
- Stories are bought from independent reporters (freelancers), press agencies such as Reuters, syndicates and members of the public
- Someone contacts the news desk of a paper or broadcasting organisation with a lead.

Features and documentaries may emerge from a topical event covered in the news, or again from the professional journals. At least one of the three or four items covered each week in Radio 4's *Medicine Now* will have come originally from a science journal such as the *British Medical Journal* or *The Health Service Journal*. Journalists working in health care scan the journals regularly for ideas and freelancers contact papers, magazines and broadcasters with ideas for features or documentaries.

Ideas also come from letters from the public and from the personal experiences of journalists and their friends and families. They can be suggested by all types of everyday experience and encounter. If a reporter has to wait in an accident and emergency unit, this may seed a feature on waiting times. If a member of a

---

Increasingly, the papers, and particularly the tabloids, are paying members of the public for first-hand accounts of events:

'A public that owns camcorders, watches Jeremy Beadle and reads every chequebook story, is getting less embarrassed and more savvy about satisfying it. 'They're more aware – more likely to pick up the phone," says [Max] Clifford, "to a paper or someone like me".'

Beckett A. (1994) I want to sell you a story. *Independent*, September 25, 1994.

Becketts' article outlines the history of some stories sold to the press, including the kidnapping of baby Abbie Humphries and the experience of a victim of necrotising fasciitis. You might like to read it. The *Independent* is available on CD-ROM

Look at some of the healthcare stories you have collected during your work on this and other Sections in the book. Can you identify their sources? You may be able to in some cases, but it is unlikely that you will be able to work out the sources of all the articles you have collected.

Some will be linked to a government report or the publication of research. If a research report is the source, can you tell whether the results have been released or leaked? If they were leaked, why might someone have been motivated to leak them? Can you tell whether the source of the research is likely to be impartial?

You may find an item that was clearly produced in response to contact by a member of the public. Can you work out the person's agenda? Has it been carried over into the report?

journalist's family has an illness which is not diagnosed for a long time, the journalist may plan an article on the condition to raise awareness of it, or of the difficulty of diagnosis. Again, coverage spawns further coverage, so if a topic is tackled in a radio broadcast, for instance, it may emerge later as the subject of a television documentary.

Who's behind the stories?

Healthcare journalists are not, as a rule, poorly-educated, elderly individuals who live in poor housing. They are generally articulate, aware of their rights, intellectual, often middle-class and white. Their range of experience is, like everyone's, limited. But this does not mean that topics likely to impact on the lives of the journalists are in general more likely to be covered than issues outside their range of experience. Good journalists and reporters have a 'nose' for stories, wherever they are and whoever is involved, and see their job as searching out the facts. There is plenty of coverage of health issues across the range of social and economic contexts.

When stories are initiated by a press release, they may be from a health authority or trust, but they may equally be from a pharmaceutical company or a research establishment. A press release from a pharmaceutical company is likely to be partial, promoting the company's products. Whether the reporter who adapts or follows up the press release is able to identify and counter bias will determine whether the final article is balanced.

Knowing the sources of an article or broadcast can alert you as reader, listener or viewer to any bias or hidden agenda. You won't always be able to identify the source of information, but when you can you need to think about:
- How the reporter has treated the source
- Whether there is any difference between what the source and the reporter aimed to get out of covering the story.

These short snippets related to medicine and health care appeared in *She*, February 1996. Items such as these may be sent in by freelancers as part of a package or put together in-house from public relations material sent to the magazine. You might like to see if you can work out the source of each item.

'A miracle birth – well, almost – has taken place in Scotland. Doctors found that a little boy they were treating had no genetic material from his father in some of his cells. It seems that he began life as a "self-activated" embryo – one that develops from an unfertilised egg. Such embryos are normally aborted early, but it seems that some of the dividing egg cells were fertilised at a later stage – allowing the baby to develop. "It's a one in a billion chance", says David Bonthron from Edinburgh University.'

'A combined calcium and magnesium liquid supplement with zinc and vitamin D might be useful for people who sweat a lot, as well as for osteoporosis, according to its makers. It costs £6.99 (inc p&p) from Salus (UK), 15 Rivington Court, Woolston Grange, Warrington, Cheshire WA1 4RT, tel: 01925 825679'

'Crossing your legs when you sit down, according to one study, increases the stability of the lower limbs and takes the stress off lower abdominal muscles, reducing fatigue.'

How a feature is written

Magazines and the newspapers print many healthcare features. They are not necessarily topical, though when an issue is currently in the news there is likely to be a flurry of features soon afterwards. Production times for some magazines make it difficult for them to follow topicality closely. A newspaper can follow up a story within a matter of days, but a monthly magazine may take two months to publish a finished article. This affects the tone as well as the content of magazine articles.

Editing and commissioning

The editor of a magazine has overall responsibility for the content. Subject editors take special responsibility for different areas. For example, health may be covered by a health and beauty editor in a magazine. On a newspaper, there may be an editor for science and medicine, or health may be grouped with social affairs or women's issues. The health editor's job is to make sure areas of health care are covered in the publication. This will probably include responsibility for particular pages or columns, and a say in the spread of coverage in the magazine or paper as a whole.

Health editors use material from in-house and freelance journalists. Freelancers may approach them with story ideas, or the editors may call someone whose work they know and ask them to write on a particular topic. The editor and journalist will agree the angle, length and deadline — which is determined by when the article is to be published. The editor may or may not want to discuss the approach the journalist is taking and be kept informed of progress. Some prefer a hands-off approach and wait for the finished article.

Producing an article

The box below outlines the path one journalist took researching and writing a story. When a journalist submits the copy (finished text) the editor reads it and approves the content, or changes it. The editor then gives it to a sub-editor who corrects the style, grammar and spelling as necessary. The sub-editor also makes cuts or changes to fit the text to the allocated space in the publication, writes headlines and subheadings and chooses the 'call-outs' (chunks of text printed in a box or other prominent position to attract attention to the story on the page). Picture researchers will come up with illustrations, sometimes guided by advice or ideas from the journalist. Finally, the sub-editor

---

Diary of a journalist

August 1995: Wrote to editor of *Cosmopolitan* with 10 stories ideas, clippings and CV.

Sept 4: Lunch with the deputy editor to discuss working on a feature about BSE. BSE was not currently in the news, having slipped out of the spotlight for a few years.

Sept 6: Received commission from deputy editor for 2500 words to be delivered in one month.

Sept 8–15: Research week. Given details of a young woman in a coma to feature as a case history. Checked the back issues of newspapers, using indices, for articles on BSE. Used the Internet for international and up-to-date sources. Read medical and science journals. Lunched with six scientists at the Medical Research Council to check the credentials of the government's critics. Got hold of government reports from the Department of Health and Ministry of Agriculture press offices, and sent a list of questions to the chief medical officer who refused to be interviewed because he was 'too busy'.

Sept 18–29: Conducted all interviews, face-to-face or over the phone. Read all reports.

Oct 2–9: Wrote first draft, revised it and sent article to two scientists for review and accuracy check. Made minor modifications and sent it to *Cosmopolitan*, by fax and on disc.

Oct 9–13: Article went to and fro between me and *Cosmopolitan* for amendments and cuts. Checked that the sub-editor's changes haven't made the article inaccurate.

Dec 95: Article published in January 1996 issue.

will pull all the elements of the article together so that it is ready for printing.

Often, the writer will not see the story after it has been accepted by the editor. Sometimes he/she may want to see it after it has been edited to check that it is still accurate and represents what she or he wanted to say. In the piece on BSE for *Cosmopolitan* cited below, both Véronique and the editor wanted to make sure that the changes the sub-editor made did not alter the sense or accuracy of the scientific material. There may be some negotiation about changes, but the editor has the final say and the writer needs a good case to stand a chance of influencing decisions.

Freelance journalists usually write for different magazines and newspapers. They may approach a publication with ideas for articles they would like to write, or they may be commissioned by editors. Preparing a story idea may require considerable research into the market. If an article is not carefully targeted to the magazine's established style and audience, it will be rejected. While writing the article on BSE which is discussed below, Véronique made sure it had human interest aspects and addressed issues that

Cosmopolitan's young female readership would be concerned with. A key element in selling the story to *Cosmopolitan* was that she knew of a young woman in a coma with Creutzfeld-Jacob Disease, the human form of spongiform encephalopathy (BSE). She feels that without this, the magazine would probably not have wanted the article.

The idea for Véronique's article came from a conversation with a scientist who expressed his concern about eating beef. Her sources included government department reports, articles in the national, medical and scientific press and interviews with scientists, representatives of medical organisations and the grandmother of Vicky Rimmer, the young girl in a coma. She had seen an item about Vicky on the TV programme *World in Action*. The producer put her in touch with Vicky's family and sent her a transcript of the programme.

Véronique spent a lot of time filtering her sources and deciding which aspects to concentrate on to make the article relevant to the target audience. She focused on three key aspects:

- The human interest of the young woman in a coma, essential for a science story
- Young women are concerned about what they eat, and many women still have responsibility for shopping for the family
- Can we trust the government?

The sub-editor cut about 500 words from the article Véronique submitted to fit it into the chosen page design and around the pictures. The cuts included most of the 'hard' scientific material. The human interest material was kept. Veronique's comment was:

'I don't like it. A story like this is built brick by brick and when you take the bricks away it's not so good.'

Find a feature article in a magazine or newspaper about a healthcare issue of which you have some knowledge or experience. Work out what sources the journalist used. You may be able to identify quotations from people interviewed, find references to reports or other written sources. Do you think the sources are reliable? Is the article accurate?

You might want to discuss your findings with others in your tutor/counsellor group. You could also build this sort of critical analysis of articles into your assessment for the unit.

How a programme is made

People rarely give a second thought to how a radio or television programme is put together. The process of orientation and interpretation in relation to the format is largely unconscious. So unless a mistake in a programme is noticed, people probably don't think about how the presenters got their information. A good programme will be seamless — you don't notice its structure or consider the process of its research and construction. This is one of the things we have come to expect of TV and is now an intrinsic part of producers' value systems. But to understand television and radio from the inside, you need to know what lies behind the piece that is broadcast.

Where does the information come from?

Producers and researchers working on radio and television programmes scan print media for ideas and information that they can use in a broadcast. They look in daily national newspapers, relevant professional and academic journals, specialist and mainstream magazines for interesting articles that may form the basis of a feature or documentary. Some regular programmes have an answerphone line for members of the public to phone in with their stories.

When a programme is planned, the producers may advertise in the *Radio Times*, newspapers and any suitable magazines for people with relevant experiences and stories to come forward. Researchers try to trace real people who have been interviewed or mentioned in the press or on other programmes. They will also call relevant professional bodies to find experts they can consult or interview. If they have found stories from members of the public through a telephone line or advertisement, these people may be interviewed or their stories used as the main interest in a feature or documentary.

Who does what?

The production team for a national radio or TV programme may be quite large. An editor (or more than one) will decide the content and angle of a programme, which features to make and whether they are of an acceptable standard. Editors also decide editorial policy, usually in line with the policy of a series or the channel. This will determine factors such as whether a programme has a political slant, is a specialised piece or should have a human interest slot, and whether it is campaigning or objective.

Diary of a radio broadcaster

Nov 4, '93: Approached producer in charge of medical items with the idea. Producer checked with programme editor before giving the go-ahead.

Nov 9: Researched subject in BBC News Information Library and BBC Subject Specialist Library.

Nov 11–16: Liaised with the press office of a centre for the treatment of stress-related facial pain. Two patients, a psychiatrist and two pyschologists agreed to be interviewed.

Nov 19: Interviewed psychiatrist, psychologist and one patient.

Nov 22: Interviewed second psychologist and second patient.

Dec 3: Copied interviews from DAT (Digital Audio Tape) to one quarter inch reel-to-reel (for editing). Digital editing on computer is gradually being introduced into radio. Noted down basic content of each interview.

Jan 5, '94: Cut tape to 12 minutes of the most interesting material. This is the rough edit.

Jan 11: Met producer to discuss rough edit.

Jan 12: Re-edited as agreed and wrote script.

Jan 18: Producer approved script then feature was recorded in a production studio. Edited clips from interviews: the sound of a therapy session and the reporter's voice were mixed together. Sound engineer edited out all the re-takes on the script. Producer edited a further minute out of the feature, and made sure it all sounded OK.

Jan 19 : Programme editor approved feature.

Feb 15: Production team for the following day's programme listened to the feature.

Feb 19: Feature broadcast.

A producer is responsible for putting the items in the broadcast together, making sure the necessary topics are covered, commissioning freelance researchers and presenters or allocating tasks to in-house staff and making sure the tapes are properly prepared. In the studio during a live broadcast, the producer is responsible for the smooth running of the programme. The producer has help from a production assistant, who may do some research and help with clerical tasks. A researcher finds the stories to cover, the information to include and the people to interview. The reporter puts the information together into a feature and may research, write and present his or her own stories. The presenter's voice is the one that is heard on the radio or television. Many features, particularly those not tied to a specific news story, are made over a period of time. Reporters are usually working on several features at once, as they often are unable to see immediately all the people they need, whether potential interviewees or busy producers.

The boxes below describe what went into a 10-minute feature on stress-related facial pain put together and broadcast by Jean Snedegar on Woman's Hour, February 16, 1994.

Woman's Hour is a one-hour programme broadcast every weekday on Radio 4. The team behind *Woman's Hour* comprises:

- Two main editors and an editor of the day
- A main presenter and occasional guest presenters
- 10 producers
- Six production assistants
- A reader, adaptor and producer for the serial
- 20–50 freelance journalists working over a month, 10–15 of whom form a team of regular contributors
- Two sound engineers a day.

A typical edition of *Woman's Hour* will include three live interviews (one or two of which may be a discussion) conducted in the studio, one in-depth feature, or two shorter features (usually called 'packages') and 13 minutes of a serialised story. The features or packages may be on healthcare topics. A 'talking point' — a live discussion in the studio — is often on a healthcare topic. A reporter may work for four or five days on a 10-minute feature for a national radio or television broadcast. Work on a feature often begins a month or more before it is due to be broadcast.

As you listen to programmes such as *You and Yours* or *Woman's Hour*, make notes on how healthcare issues are presented. How many experts are interviewed? How many patients or other 'real people'? What is the angle taken?

Arrange with others in your tutor/counsellor group to watch two programmes such as *Panorama*, *Horizon*, *Despatches*, or *Public Eye* on a healthcare topic. Discuss the coverage of the issues raised and the editorial policy. You may get ideas for your assessment for the unit from this Activity.

Conclusion

This Section started by looking at two theoretical strands which offer widely differing perspectives on media:

- Dominance theory — the idea that a dominant ideology pervades the media and helps to assert what Marxists call the 'cultural hegemony' of middle class values
- Pluralist theory — the idea that different groups in society are represented in the media and that no single ideology prevails (Abercrombie, 1980); this idea links to the interpretative reading of media and post-modernist descriptions of the way people create their own identities.

The media are not immune to influence — from inside (owners, boards) and outside (government, pressure groups). Because they come from different directions, these pressures may play a balancing role in themselves, helping the media to reflect a diverse range of opinion. Commercial pressures through advertising are powerful, but even here the argument runs that advertisements reflect the desires of consumers and so match the economic priorities of society. Even advertisements themselves are 'codes' which people interpret in the light of their own constructions of reality — people do not obey a simple trigger-response rule in relation to media messages.

The Section then looked at some of the constraints on the way the mass media constructs its own self-identity through the mix of stories in newspapers and the way they are written, the flow of programmes on TV or radio. Once again, there is room for opposing viewpoints. Does the disciplined, co-ordinated activity needed to bring out a daily paper or produce a programme on radio or TV suggest a common purpose, which at the level of the whole network supports a particular view of society? Or is the chaos of the newsroom or studio evidence of a multiplicity of separate purposes?

References

Abercrombie, N., Hill, S. and Turner, B. (1980) *The Dominant Ideology Thesis*. London: Allen and Unwin.

Barthes, R. The photographic message. In: Sontag, S. (ed.) (1993) *A Roland Barthes Reader*. London: Vintage.

Dennett, H.D. (1991) *Consciousness Explained*. London: Penguin.

Eco, U. (1995) *Apocalypse Postponed*. London: HarperCollins.

Giddens, A. (1986) *The Constitution of Society*. London: Polity Press.

Illich, I. (1972) *Deschooling Society*. London: M. Boyars.

McLuhan, M. (1964) *Understanding Media: The extensions of man*. London: Routledge. (Reprinted 1994.)

McQuail, D. (1987) *Mass Communication Theory: An introduction* London: Sage Publications (second edition).

Philo, G. (1995) Television, politics and the rise of the new right. In: Philo, G. (ed). *Glasgow Media Group Reader. Volume 2*. London: Routledge.

Thompson, E.P. (1968) *The Making of the English Working Class*. Harmondsworth: Penguin.

Williams, R. (1975) *Television: Technology and cultural form*. (Revised 1990.) London: Routledge.

Look back at the analysis of the media you have carried out so far in this unit.

Which aspects of your analysis tend to support a dominant ideology and which a pluralist theory?

How do your ideas about the media link in with your ideas about society?

'Network is often used, unfortunately, to designate the channels reserved to materials selected by others for indoctrination, instruction or entertainment. But it can also be used for the telephone or postal service, which are primarily accessible to individuals who want to send messages to each other. I wish we had another word to designate such reticular structures for mutual access, a word less evocative of entrapment...'

Illich, I. (1972) *Deschooling Society*. London: M, Boyars.

Introduction

This Section looks at how public demand and the constraints of production interact on the media. It focuses on:
- Types of media — forms of printed and broadcast media which are likely to carry healthcare coverage (pages 62–73)
- Issues of content — the ways in which health care is represented, and the type of topic that comes up in different forms of media (pages 74–83).

The interplay of technical, practical and social factors means that we receive different kinds of messages from the different media. As you investigate different forms of the media in this Section, bear in mind the different ways in which they mediate experiences: reading a description of someone is not the same as seeing a picture of that person; watching a video of someone is not the same as meeting the person.

Keep asking yourself what your own role is in constructing the message you get from the media. Work out how your role changes between different media (broadcast and print) and between different products in the same medium. For example, is your role the same as a reader of the *Guardian* as when you are a reader of the *Sun*?

How do you respond to these different forms of the same product? For example, if you read a report in a newspaper you dislike and don't trust, do you discount what it says ('What can you expect...?') and do you respond emotionally to what seems like unfair or inaccurate reporting? When you read reports of the same story in a paper you like and trust, do you believe it is true? And do you still respond emotionally? ('Have you read this? It's terrible...').

Pick a topical healthcare story. Compare the treatment of the story you have picked in different media. What differences are there related to the form rather than the particular characteristics of the programme or publication? Make notes in your learning journal on how the story is presented in different media, and your response to its presentation. Can you explain and account for how it affects you differently?

'Citizens must be able to rely on a free, an independent and a diversified press to inform them clearly about the facts essential to an understanding of the problems and advise them, from various points of view, of the solutions.'

Lord Shawcross, Chairman of the Press Council, 1974. Quoted in: Best, G., Dennis, J. and Draper, P. (1977) *Health, the Mass Media and the National Health Service.* London: Unit for the Study of Health Policy.

When did they start?	
Times	1785
Observer	1791
Guardian	1821
Sunday Times	1822
The Daily Telegraph	1855
People	1881
Daily Mail	1896
Daily Express	1900
Daily Mirror	1903
Sun	1969
BBC	1922 (incorporated 1927)
BBC News	1926
BBC1	1946
ITV	1954
BBC2	1962
Channel 4	1982
Channel 5	1987

Commercial TV and the BBC

When the BBC was incorporated in 1927 it was envisaged as a provider of public service broadcasting. Its characteristic attitude over the next few decades was as a paternalistic, moral guardian of the people. It took it upon itself to educate, improve and direct the choice of its listeners and, later, viewers. John Reith, who was in charge of the Corporation from its inception, rejected audience research: he did not want to pander to the tastes of the public, but to dictate and improve them. This attitude eventually gave way in the face of competition, both from within the BBC as more services were set up, and from independent television (ITV). Recently, cable and satellite service-providers have added to the competition.

Television channels compete for viewers, therefore competition dictates the content and timing of programmes. Broadcasters soon found that if one channel broadcast a documentary while the other broadcast light entertainment, the viewing figures for the documentary were low. So they both broadcast their documentaries at the same time, maximising viewing figures for the genre. As Reith said: 'It does not matter how many thousands there may be listening: there is always enough for others'.

Commercialism and quality

'Commercial television produces audiences not programmes' (Curran and Seaton, 1991). If this is the case, who are the consumers of television? Advertisers or viewers? Independent television has to attract viewers to make its advertising attractive. If there are few viewers, the advertising time is not worth much. The BBC has to attract viewers to justify its licence fee. However the BBC can subsidise quality programming which may attract fewer viewers. Some of these programmes, such as costume drama, earn their keep from foreign sales. Other areas, such as high-quality current affairs and documentaries, add to the BBC's prestige — its cultural capital rather than its bank account.

Commercial pressures affect what is broadcast, but the BBC is guided to some extent by its charter and the ITC enforces a framework of regulations designed to control the output of independent television. The aim is to maintain balanced programming and 'due impartiality', and also to make sure that television does not turn into a feast of uninterrupted gameshows and repeated soap operas. In order to keep their franchises, the independent television companies have to comply with the requirements of the

A 'home' programme would 'be generally so designed that it will steadily, but imperceptibly, raise the standard of taste, entertainment, outlook and citizenship.'

BBC Internal Memorandum (1944) 'Programme development.' London: BBC Written Archives, February 14, 1944. Quoted in: Curran, J. and Seaton, J. (1991) *Power Without Responsibility: The press and broadcasting in Britain*. London: Routledge (4th edition).

'Commercial television is a very unusual business...you don't necessarily make more money if you provide a better product.'

Sidney Bernstein, quoted in: Curran, J. and Seaton, J. (1991) *Power without Responsibility: The press and broadcasting in Britain*. London: Routledge (4th edition), p232.

Different researchers have come up with opposing findings about people's viewing behaviour. Some find that viewers are indiscriminate — they will not necessarily watch programmes of a particular type, consecutive episodes of a serial or the same channel consistently. Others find that viewers are most affected by content — they choose programmes they are interested in and watch those.

Monitor your own viewing habits over two or three weeks. Do you turn on and watch whatever comes along, or choose your viewing selectively? If you do both, what makes you more likely to do one or the other? Examine the mental processes that go on as a result of watching TV. Do you simply accept the rapid flickering of content and presentation from one programme to another? Or does your mind make an attempt to integrate the fragmentary culture of the post-modern TV experience?

ITC, and to be financially successful they have to attract advertisers by making their programmes attractive to the right number and type of viewers.

Audience profiles

Advertisers want their advertisements to be seen by people who may buy their product or service. Many of the products advertised on television are targeted at young people and couples. To attract advertisers, programming is geared towards attracting these types of viewers. This affects scheduling (when a particular programme is shown) and editorial content. For example, documentaries tend to concentrate on personal and human interest stories and case histories, as women have been found to like this. Morning television has a magazine format because it is directed mostly at people who are able to watch during the day, which may include unemployed and older people as well as the traditional audience of women.

Audiences for other types of programmes are more socially wide-ranging, which makes it difficult for advertisers to target likely consumers. But the growth of programmes (and cable and satellite channels) relating to special interests such as travel, motoring and gardening, makes it easier for advertisers to time their advertisements for maximum relevant exposure. This in turn affects scheduling.

Independent television companies are allowed to broadcast up to seven minutes of 'spot' advertising an hour (advertisements in commercial breaks). Since 1988, sponsorship of programmes has also been allowed to defray the cost of producting a programme, although news broadcasts may not be sponsored. The producer of a sponsored programme has to make sure it is good enough to attract many viewers so that the sponsor's investment pays off.

How is it possible to tell what difference, if any, commercial considerations make to the quality of programmes on BBC and independent television? How could you find out if the cost-conscious, managerial culture of the BBC is likely to produce different results from the profit-oriented ethos of the independent TV franchise holders?

Advertisers buy time on television either in the form of guaranteed viewing figures, or as particular slots. Guaranteed figures will probably consist of some prime-time slots and some less popular slots. Particular slots are chosen with regard to the schedules, published quarterly in advance. Advertisers try to place commercials near programmes that will enhance their product or bring a favourable response to it. They try to avoid slots that will reduce the effect of their advertisements. Thus Sainsbury's may advertise after a food programme, but British Airways is unlikely to advertise after a documentary on air crashes.

If you are interested in the commercial influences on television programming, draw a spider diagram to show the interlocking interests that affect what is broadcast.

'I had a presentiment that the "travelling" phase of my life might be passing. I felt, before the malaise of settlement crept over me, that I should...set down on paper a résumé of the ideas, quotations and encounters which had amused and obsessed me; and which I hoped would shed light on what is, for me, the question of questions: the nature of human restlessness.'

Chatwin, B. (1987) *The Songlines*. London: Pan Books Ltd.

How would you portray yourself in relation to your investigation of the media? Are you an explorer setting out to chart the territory or do you see yourself more as a wanderer?

National newspapers

National newspapers are divided into tabloids and broadsheets (also called the quality press), catering for different markets.

Format and price

Tabloids are small-format newspapers (16in. x 23in.) conventionally considered to be down-market. They have a high proportion of images to text and a colloquial, familiar style of writing. They carry less serious news than the broadsheets, and tend towards coverage of human interest stories. Their reporting of events, even serious news events, has a human interest slant. There is a strong tendency towards sensationalism. The cover price is generally low therefore the circulation has to be high for a paper to succeed. A greater proportion of the revenue from a tabloid paper comes from the cover price than from advertising.

A broadsheet newspaper is double the size of a tabloid. Some have a tabloid pull-out section. They have a high proportion of text, a more formal tone than the tabloids, use more complex grammar and a wider vocabulary. The cover price of a broadsheet can be higher than that of a tabloid, but in the circulation wars of the early 1990s the price of the *Times* and *The Daily Telegraph* fell to tabloid levels. A greater proportion of the revenue from a broadsheet comes from the advertising it carries than from its cover price.

The weekend quality papers, and particularly the Sundays, come with a large number of supplements catering for different areas of interest, such as arts, sport, business and news analysis. Some have a tabloid and some a magazine format. The Sundays blur the boundaries between newspapers, which traditionally concentrate on the topical, and magazines, which carry more reflective and non-topical material. They also open up new possibilities in advertising sales.

Ownership and political bias

Most national newspapers are owned by a few very large corporations, which often have other media interests and holdings in other types of companies. Because several titles are owned by the same organisation, there is apparently competition within the holdings of a single organisation. On the whole, though, these titles are not in direct competition with each other as the papers are quite different. For example, News International, which owns the *Times* and *Sun*, has

---

'Larry Lamb, first editor of the *Sun* under Murdoch's proprietorship, said that "newspapers had to be designed for the gratification of readers, not journalists...The only reliable measure of a newspaper's quality was not the opinion of journalists and critics, but the number of people who bought it."'

Chippindale, P. and Horrie, C. (1990) *Stick it Up Your Punter*. London: Heinneman.

'We are occasionally guilty of being indiscriminate in the use of extreme terms to describe a situation, but we are a tabloid newspaper. We are obliged to use a form of journalistic shorthand to give punch and emphasis to news stories.'

Kenneth Donlan of the *Sun*, quoted In: Vousden, M. (1985) 'Loony lefties' and 'mad mullahs'. *Nursing Times* 85: 28: 16-17.

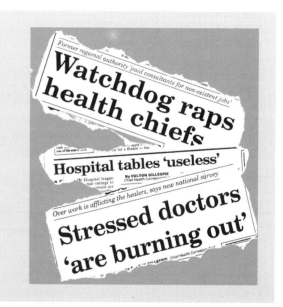

papers at opposite ends of the market. News International can try to maximise its total share of the market by promoting both an up-market paper and a down-market paper, knowing that there is little danger of poaching its own readers.

National and regional papers tend to support one political party — more support the Conservatives than Labour or other parties. This broad tendency disguises a more complex picture, especially in relation to the way people vote or think politically. Labels don't help very much here. The *Sun* is not a progressive or left-wing paper. But many *Sun* readers vote Labour and one of the paper's editorial policies is to attack the Royal Family, not normally a conservative position. It may be more useful to think of the distinctive character of the paper — populist and forthright — as forming a bond with readers, rather than its political allegiance. The *Express* may sell itself as the voice of a Tory government, but the paper supports a particular brand of Conservatism and may sometimes attack both the policies and individual members of the government. The *Guardian* is read mainly by left-wing people but it is often critical of the Labour party and its readership traverses a wide range of political allegiance, from Liberal

Democrat to Green and alternative politics. Newspapers which try to be politically independent, such as the *Independent*, often create a compliance that is anti-political, leaving the reader with a feeling that there is little to choose between political parties.

The most important thing to remember with the press, as with other media, is that people form their own relationship with newspapers. They get to know some very well and anticipate their voice as they do the voices of people they know, making allowances here and approving there. Other newspapers remain more or less unknown, unsympathetic in allegiance and alien in character.

Healthcare coverage
Healthcare news is covered by both tabloids and broadsheets, though the broadsheets will generally give fuller coverage, with analysis and comment based on political, ethical and economic criteria. Broadsheets have editors or correspondents assigned to dealing with health and medical issues. They are responsible for ensuring adequate, accurate and fair coverage of these issues. There will sometimes be reflective or analytical articles about health care. Comment in the tabloids is likely to be human-interest based.

Buy a copy of a tabloid and a broadsheet newspaper on the same day. Make a chart or a table to itemise the differences between them. Look at layout, content, tone and style of writing, bias, price, advertising, reader offers and any other features that interest you. You might want to discuss your findings with others in your tutor/counsellor group.

It is quite an interesting exercise to look at an unfamiliar newspaper and see how long it takes you to orientate yourself to its layout, political allegiances and — more difficult — its distinctive character. The differences from what you are used to can be even greater with a foreign paper. Try it with a paper such as the *International Herald Tribune*, written in the United States mainly for the expatriate American market, though read more widely.

These newspapers have on-line versions which can be accessed over the Internet on the World Wide Web:

The Daily Telegraph
http://www.telegraph.co.uk (started 1995)

Guardian
http://www.guardian.co.uk (started 1995)

The Times
http://www.the-times.co.uk (started 1996)

If you would like to know more about the history of newspaper publishing in the UK, read:

Curran, J. and Seaton, J. (1991) *Power without Responsibility: The press and broadcasting in Britain*. London: Routledge (4th edition).

Ingham, B. (1991) *Kill the Messenger*. London: HarperCollins (hardback). London: Fontana (softback).

Chippindale, P. and Horrie, C. (1990) *Stick it Up Your Punter*. London: Heinemann.

Local papers, TV and radio

It is easy to underestimate the importance of the local media and to concentrate on national TV, radio and press. But the local press is an important source of information. The total circulation of paid-for local papers, daily and weekly, is around 18 million and of free local papers, around 37 million. The total circulation of the national daily press is around 14 million.

The local press is usually the most important source of information about local healthcare services, hospital trusts and local politics which may have an impact on health issues for a large portion of the population. It also has a powerful effect on how people view the quality and availability of health care locally. For example, when a ward shuts or a patient dies in controversial circumstances, reporters may write critical stories about the service generally or specific clinical and/or management decisions that were made. For these reasons, trusts have press officers whose job it is to form good relations with the local media, get positive coverage and provide a channel for healthcare professionals and managers to communicate with the media (see pages 106–107 and 114–115).

National press and broadcasting often pick up stories from local papers. The items may then become national news stories, or bring new issues onto the political agenda. A story may move from the local to the national arena because someone working for a national organisation spots it. More often, reporters on local papers feed stories directly to the nationals. Most reporters working on local papers aspire to working on the nationals and are keen to get their stories taken up to maximise their own exposure: 'Local stories can, by this route, structure national news agendas. This happened when a Birmingham hospital was unable to perform very urgent and necessary heart surgery on young children because of a shortage of resources. After a number of airings in the local media, the story contributed substantially to making the hospital crisis a national news story which ran throughout the winter of 1987 to1988' (Franklin and Murphy, 1991).

Local papers

Local papers can span a diverse range of opinion. Many express sympathy for causes such as homelessness and unemployment that are given less detailed treatment in the nationals. This is partly because there is more diversity in

What features of the story reprinted here made it attractive to the national media?

'Hospital's abortion mix-up

'A mother had a healthy baby aborted after being mistakenly told it had Down's syndrome by Addenbrooke's Hospital, it was revealed today.

'The tragedy occurred when two samples from West Suffolk health district got mixed up at the hospital's cytogenetics laboratory. The samples had been sent there for routine analysis and, during the testing process, had been wrongly labelled.

'The mistake led to a mother with a Down's syndrome baby being told it was all right, and the mother with the healthy baby... having an abortion.'

Cambridge Evening News, November 6, 1995

The editor of the *Cambridge Evening News* which printed the story reproduced in the adjacent column, later reflected on the relationship between trusts and newspaper reporting: 'Since trusts were set up they have been run like company boards. A lot of the members are business people who are not used to doing something in public. But the more done in public, the more the public will feel involved with that authority and support its activities.'

Eaton, L. (1997) What the papers say. *Health Service Journal*. 107: January 9.

First local BBC radio station	1967
First local independent radio station	1972
Cable Authority established	1985

ownership of these papers, although more and more local papers are now owned by large groups and syndicates. A more important reason is the need to build up local sympathy and a feeling of solidarity in order to protect and build circulation: the local press must speak with a voice sympathetic to local opinion on local matters.

The local paper is widely seen as the accessible part of the media, and often the first line of attack for a member of the public who wants to get something changed is to write to the local paper. It may be a letter for the letters page, or to suggest an investigative or news article. However, letters do not need always to be a response to an article published in the paper: they can introduce a new topic, and open up channels for discussion. They can also initiate change as a result of mobilising local public opinion. In fund-raising for hospitals, the local press is a particularly powerful way of reaching local people who will be concerned enough to give and raise money.

Local broadcasting

Local radio and television are divided into BBC regional radio and television and the independent local stations. Independents include franchised regional broadcasters and the new cable channels which make community television a real possibility for the near future, even though cable TV can be watched only by those with appropriate cabling and is more expensive to set up. Local radio can be on a very small scale — right down to the hospital's own radio service. This would not be feasible for television at the moment.

As national news coverage becomes more international in focus, the role of the local broadcast media as providers of relevant news becomes more crucial. People can be just as worried about ward closures at their local hospital — which may impinge directly on their lives — as about issues such as national funding for mental health provision which may affect them only indirectly, if at all. The local press often campaign against change. Public opinion is mobilised against, say, the closure of a local accident and emergency department, without necessarily considering the benefits of having specialised centres elsewhere in the region.

Independent television is divided into franchises for different geographic regions of the country. The regions are not equal in power, population or wealth. The network is dominated by programmes made by the most lucrative franchises. Some regions, such as London, can afford to make expensive programmes, depending on high-value advertising and syndicating the programmes to recoup costs. The smaller or poorer regions can make fewer of their own programmes and can afford to make costly programmes only if they can guarantee network sales. This means that although regional television franchises could apparently have led to good local television, they have actually led to the poorer regions buying in more programmes. The quality drops to cut costs.

Where people get their local news:

TV	19%
Radio	12%
Papers	56%
Other people	9%

Franklin, B. and Murphy, D. (1991) *What News? The market, politics and the local press.* London: Routledge.

Ask half a dozen friends, relatives or colleagues to find out what local media they use. To what extent do they watch local TV news, listen to local radio, buy a local paper, read the local free sheets? How does this relate to what they see and read in the national media?

You might like to extend this into a proper survey, or analyse your own use of the national and local media over a period of, say, a month. What might be the significance of your findings to the work of healthcare professionals?

Professional journals

One source of healthcare coverage, which you are likely to use yourself, is the professional journals. These are also a source for other areas of the media. Producers and reporters who specialise in healthcare coverage scan relevant journals such as the *Lancet*, *BMJ*, *The Health Service Journal* and *Nursing Times* looking for new stories or new angles on existing stories. Looking back at the coverage of an issue in professional journals after it has been covered in the mass media can give you an insight into how a topic is picked up, how the material is selected and how emphasis may be added or changed.

Professional journals are aimed at an audience of practitioners. They assume a certain amount of knowledge — of healthcare or medical issues, specialist vocabulary, research traditions and methods and the context of the journal itself. A lay reader coming to the *Lancet* may find much of interest, but also much that is obscure or relates to debates in the academic or professional press.

Professional journals are edited by professionals. They reflect the views of the profession, or part of it — *Nursing Standard* is owned by the RCN, the main nursing union; *Nursing Times* calls itself 'The independent voice of nursing' and aims at unbiased coverage. These 'popular' journals contain up-to-date information about issues and practice; they can lobby (for example the *Nursing Times* campaign in 1995 for 3% for nurses), they are a source of jobs and they can campaign on behalf of patients/clients (for example, the campaign in 1996 in *Nursing Times* for older people — 'Elderly Care Counts'). Popular journals are complemented by more scholarly journals such as the *Journal of Advanced Nursing*. Both types of journal 'have played a particularly valuable role in recent decades by reorienting nurses away from the dominance of medical and social science models of nursing, to a more appropriate nursing orientation' (Smith, 1996).

Accuracy and reliability

Professional journals provide a forum for research carried out by healthcare professionals. Often, articles are the result of months or years of painstaking research. They may have been subject to peer review; this means that the editor has asked other experts to read an article and assess the quality of the research and the interpretation of results. Although the reviewers do not repeat the research, they look critically at

---

The core degree unit, *Enquiring into Healthcare Practice*, contains a great deal of information and good practice on how to plan, set up and carry out a practice-based research or enquiry project. If you are particularly interested in media issues, this book may suggest ideas for your own enquiry-based project.

Writers in professional journals may use jargon to:

- Convey precise meaning
- Defuse emotional issues: it is emotionally easier to read about 'perinatal mortality' than about 'babies who die'
- Validate professionals' elite knowledge
- Exclude non-professional readers.

Examine your own reading of professional journals as a practitioner.

Which professional journals do you read regularly?

How often do you read them?

Why do you read these journals and not others?

What sorts of articles do you like to read in them?

Which other journals would you be interested to read in future?

What are the influences and pressures that make professional journals more circumspect than a national newspaper?

the methods and the conduct of it. Research reports aim to be objective, but it is often difficult to avoid some subjectivity in interpreting results. Researchers often begin with a hypothesis they want to test, or at least with some idea of the type of results they expect to find. It is all too easy to interpret the results in the light of the hypothesis or expectations, even if these eventually turn out to have been misguided or irrelevant. So although the research may have been conducted rigorously using valid methods, the evaluation of the results may still be debatable. For example, if a nurse researcher found that patients recovered more quickly if nurses spent less time talking socially with them, she would be likely to try to interpret the results differently, or look for another factor, to avoid drawing the conclusion that social conversation with patients slows their recovery. This is a completely hypothetical case, but it shows how a researcher's bias can direct the interpretation of results.

The voice of reason

The 'voice' of articles in professional journals can be authoritative, dispassionate and seemingly non-partisan. The tendency is to make it look as though the research speaks for itself,

and the role of interpretation is often minimised. These features can combine to make the articles persuasive and transparent: readers cannot see the article as a construct, only the 'facts' it reports. You may have to train yourself to reflect on articles in journals rather than swallow them wholesale. Here are some tips for critical reading:

- Look at who carried out the research — do they have the right sort of experience?
- Think about the methods that have been used, the choice of sample, the interpretation of the results.
- Even when the article does not invite you to think critically, make a habit of doing so.
- Do not be taken in by the voice just because it sounds authoritative. After all, if an issue was certain, it would not be the subject of research in the first place, so be alert to the possibility of faulty methods, inaccuracy and misguided interpretation.

A research article in a professional journal generally presents all details of the methods, then the results, then the interpretation of them. It may include an explanation of choices made, extra validation, checks and so on. Most of this material will be dropped if the article moves into the mainstream media that most people see.

An article in *Nature* (December 29, 1995) on BSE contained details which indicated that research suggesting that BSE could not be transmitted to humans was flawed: the researchers had not waited for the full incubation period and had only looked at the presence of one of the necessary proteins. The coverage in the mass media presented the findings as fact with no qualification.

'It is a sign of professional and intellectual immaturity to assume that being popular and being serious are incompatible, or that opinions dressed up in research trappings are the only ones worth noting...Mimicking the scholarly journals means we could alienate the vast majority of our readers — precisely those who rarely read research, who are not in academic institutions and who are the people we most need to influence when it comes to improving nursing.'

Jane Salvage, editor of *Nursing Times* (personal communication to the editor of the *Journal of Advanced Nursing*, July 1996).

General interest magazines

There are magazines and programmes for most groups in society. Healthcare coverage constitutes a variable proportion of their content, but is important in many. What type of healthcare information and advice do people get from these magazines, and what is its role? To answer these questions it is also necessary to ask questions at a broader level about the nature of these magazines and the strategies readers have for decoding and interpreting them.

Women's magazines

The average circulation of the top eight women's monthlies in the first half of 1996 was 2.1 million. Their main purpose is to entertain and they are not educational texts in the same way as professional journals. But health has become big business, so the recipes are promoted as 'healthy', the problem page offers solutions to problems such as stress and many of the magazines contain a regular feature on new health-related products.

Women's magazines are the largest sector of the magazine market and a source of information on health and fitness for many women. Split broadly into the quality monthlies and the more down-market weeklies, they contain coverage of women's and children's health issues, but often also of issues relating specifically to men (prostate problems, testicular cancer, and so on). In contrast to men's magazines, which focus on health for men, women's magazines recognise that women generally take responsibility for health within the family

Apart form the explicit coverage of healthcare issues, women's magazines have an impact on their readers' body image and perceptions of what it is to be healthy and beautiful. They frequently group together health and beauty on the contents page and articles on these subjects may be the responsibility of a 'health and beauty' editor. A healthy diet and an exercise régime are often promoted as a means of attaining a 'desirable' body rather than as valuable targets in their own right. Health and beauty magazines such as *Top Santé* do not distinguish at all between being healthy and being beautiful. Although they may pay lip-service to weight loss as an aid to health, the thrust is clearly towards the 'thin is beautiful' model of perfection. As a result, women who are dissatisfied with their physical appearance may feel not only that they are not attractive, but also that they are not healthy.

Get hold of a women's weekly such as *Woman's Realm*, *Woman*, *Bella*,or *Best*, and one monthly such as *She*, *Options*, or *Cosmopolitan*.Cut out or mark all the healthcare items and decide which of these four categories they fall into:

- Medical — focusing on conventional treatment, medical advances, hospital procedures
- 'Help yourself' — what individuals can do to promote health, including dealing with illness, healthy living, diet and preventive measures
- Consumerism — the patient as healthcare consumer, covering rights, choices and taking responsibility for treatment
- Environmental — how environmental and social factors affect health and well-being.

Is there a noticeable difference in the degree of coverage the weekly and monthly magazines give each aspect?

An article in the magazine *Top Santé* about sick building syndrome aimed to dispel people's feelings of disempowerment by suggesting what readers could do to minimise the effects of an unhealthy building. Just pointing out the problems with poorly-designed buildings may have affected readers in different ways:

- Enrage them, so that they press for action
- Undermine their confidence — they feel the issue is out of their control
- Worry them — they feel they can't do anything, but are being affected by their environment. The worry is likely to add to any problems.

By making suggestions, the article avoided a wholly environmental approach, empowered its readers and may perhaps have prompted them to correct environmental conditions. But does this sort of approach also shift responsibility away from architects, builders and building managers onto individuals?

Images on reality

The images of youth, health, beauty and lifestyle that predominate in women's magazines do not reflect the reality of most women's lives, but these magazines are read by a large cross-section of the population. It is a sophisticated sort of reading, in which the ideals portrayed by the magazine are discounted against the reality. Something may be retained that can be of use or value in real life: one feminist view is that these images are part of the 'cultural management of female desire and female flight from a purely reproductive destiny' (Winckler, 1994). But the cumulative effect may be what psychoanalysts call 'narcissistic injury': the preoccupation with fat, diet, exercise and the perfect body may 'function as one of the most powerful normalizing strategies of our century... [producing] bodies habituated to self-discipline and self-improvement' (Bardo, 1990).

Men's magazines

Ask men what types of magazine they read and you might hear a catalogue of car, motorbike, computer and sporting titles. Some may mention 'top shelf', soft porn titles if they are willing to admit to reading them. But men's magazines such as *GQ*, *FM* or *Loaded* (the market leader) are a growing sector of the magazine market. The average circulation of the top seven men's magazines in the first half of 1996 was just under one million. They resemble women's magazines in many ways, carrying healthcare coverage along with style, politics and general current affairs articles. Magazines of this type are usually bought by young, professional men with above average income. Their health coverage focuses mostly on male health issues such as impotence, other types of sexual dysfunction, depression and mental illness. As with women's magazines, there is a confusion between health/fitness and attractiveness. A similar sort of sophisticated reading is required in which each reader assesses the images against his own reality.

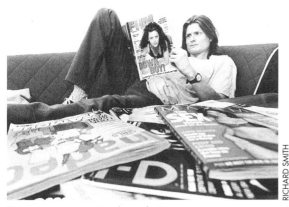

RICHARD SMITH

'...men are pretty simple souls.'

Ask yourself the question: 'Who (if anyone) is being exploited by the health-related issues in general magazines?' Is it wrong to have healthy recipes just because they sell magazines? Is it right to inform people about products which claim to improve health? Are the messages about healthy lifestyles likely to encourage readers to live in a more healthy way?

Buy a copy of a men's magazine, such as *GQ* or *Men's Health*. Look at the articles and illustrations and identify the ways in which they promote health. How are they different from articles and illustrations in women's magazines?

Do you think men's magazines do or could help promote health care? Could they use some of the methods you use in your dealings with male patients/clients, or could you adopt any of their methods?

'All we did is get back to basics and acknowledge that men are pretty simple souls.'

Alan Lewis, editor of *Loaded*. Quoted in: Glaister, D. (1996) Now it's lads on top. *Guardian*, August, 5 1996.

On-line media

Traditional published and broadcast media are not the only media from which people get information about healthcare issues. People are now using electronic information services such as the Internet to get their news and exchange views with others. About one million people in the UK have access to these services, drawn disproportionately from the professional and managerial classes. In some geographic areas, it is likely that more patients than healthcare practitioners will have access to healthcare information on the Internet (Coiera, 1996). As with traditional media, these privileged people may have a disproportionate influence on the way issues are reflected in the new media.

The Internet

The most important forms of communications on the Internet are:

- Electronic mail (e-mail)
- Bulletin boards
- On-line publishing: the World Wide Web.

Messages can be sent and received in the form of e-mail or bulletin board postings. These are usually just text but can include sound, pictures and video clips. Most e-mail is 'person to person', but it is also possible to set up mailing lists: a single message is then sent to many people. This can be one way, as for an electronic newsletter, or two-way, where each reader can reply and create a discussion. As well as e-mail and mailing lists, which are largely private, there are also on-line bulletin boards. These are just like the poster boards in hospital corridors: anyone can post a message and anyone can read it. On-line publications are probably the most important as a source of discussion of healthcare issues, followed by bulletin boards.

The Internet gives access to a massive on-line library through the World Wide Web. Millions of documents are available on the Web; you can display, print and search them. The Web is at the centre of a revolution in the way the publishing industry works. Newspapers such as the *Guardian, Times* and *The Daily Telegraph* are all now publishing on-line editions, as are many professional journals such as the *BMJ* (http://www.bmj.com/bmj). The BBC has a large presence on the World Wide Web, and uses it to provide background information and programme support material, as does Channel 4. The Internet is an interactive medium: people expect to use it to comment and discuss issues. When a major healthcare topic comes up, it will

The unit *Health Care and the Information Age* has more information on how healthcare professionals, patients and clients are using electronic media. If you are new to the Internet, you might like to read:

Pallen, M. (1995) Introducing the Internet. *BMJ* 311: 1422-4.

What is the advantage of being able to access information about health care across the world? What can healthcare professionals do with all this information to improve their practice and extend their view of the world?

What possible problems are there? For example, it may feel less comfortable reading material on screen rather than on a page. Or the cultural differences between one approach to health care and another may set up barriers or lead to confusion.

If you have access to the Internet or an on-line service, look for a discussion group concerned with health care. It might be a professional discussion group, or a self-help group. Read the current messages and see how much information is given. Check the facts given against other sources. Would you have faith in the advice coming from these sources?

'Mass media people have read McLuhan too late. The present and the forthcoming young generation is and will be a computer-oriented generation. The main feature of a computer screen is that it hosts and displays more alphabetic letters than images. The new generation will be alphabet and not image-oriented.'

Eco, U. (1995) The future of literacy. In: *Apocalypse Postponed*. London: HarperCollins.

permeate all areas of the network. The Internet is also international: advice or information can be sought from around the world. This may be helpful but it can also be misleading, since healthcare practice is different in other countries.

Quality and control

It is much easier to put information out on the Internet than it is to get time on a national TV programme or space in a professional journal. But much of the information and comment is opinionated, inaccurate and could be dangerous: the Internet is still very much a public forum for debate, and while an increasing number of professional news organisations are using it, there is no guarantee of quality just because something is well produced. On-line publication also highlights the issues of objectivity and perspective — with no obvious solution in sight. The organised medical networked information (OMNI) initiative gives guidance on the best available sources of healthcare information (http://www.omni.cot.ac.uk).

There is debate about how to protect children from accessing inappropriate material on the Net. This is affecting the coverage of health care. For example, in late 1995, America OnLine removed all of its chat areas that had the word 'breast' in them in an attempt to stifle pornography. However, the women running breast cancer support groups on-line complained, and the groups have since been reinstated. At about the same time, CompuServe withdrew access to a number of Internet discussion groups from its subscribers because it was threatened with prosecution in Germany. Among the groups withdrawn were several offering support and counselling to gays and lesbians. As another example, an amendment to the US Telecommunications Act prohibits the use of computer networks to transmit 'offensive or indecent' messages; this could easily include discussion of health issues. Because health care covers such a wide range of areas, many of which are potentially embarrassing, there is a real danger that, inadvertently, healthcare material will be censored.

The Department of Health has a site on the web (http://www.open.gov.uk/doh/dhhome.html) where it has made available a range of information, including *The Health of the Nation*. There are very many health-related discussion groups and mailing lists. The following are some of those listed at the Good Health Web (http://www.social.com/health/index.html):

alt.med.allergy — helping people with allergies
misc.health.aids — general discussion of AIDS/HIV
misc.health.arthritis
sci.med — information about medical products and regulations
sci.med.nursing — questions and talk about nursing
alt.support.arthritis
alt.support.asthma
alt.support.cancer
alt.support.sinusitis
AUTISM SJU — autism and developmental disabilities list
BREAST-CANCER — breast cancer discussion list
DIET - support and discussion of weight loss
DOWN-SYN — Down's syndrome
DRUGABUS — drug abuse education information and research

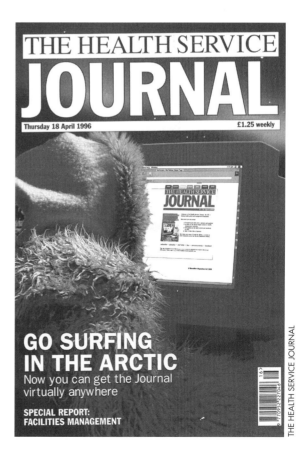

Shock – horror – probe

Sensational headlines are meant to make you stop and look. To make a story more sensational, a publication or programme may play on existing fears, or call up resonances and associations which will instil fear or horror. This may be very subtle, such as using a particular type of photograph which recalls a famous image, or overt, such as likening an epidemic to the Black Death. Emotive words may also be used in the headline and copy: a headline such as 'Beds cuts shock' tells us to be shocked, while 'Brave Kelly's fight against hospital red tape' implies it.

Sensationalist healthcare coverage tends to focus on scares, epidemics, particularly horrific individual personal experiences of illness or injury and the psychology of crime (closely allied to crime reporting). If the issue is too distant, its effect is reduced. If taken too far, it can produce panic. The most sensational stories threaten some sort of social disorder. But panic may have far-reaching social consequences which can be detrimental and may rebound in the form of criticism of the media (Karpf, 1988). Stories from other countries such as those reporting on Ebola fever in 1995 and the outbreak of bubonic plague in India in 1994, needed to emphasise

the high death rate, provide gory details and imply a threat to the UK to have maximum impact. In both these cases, the danger of the disease being brought to Britain by travellers was exaggerated by the media because it was not really a significant risk, but it gave a dimension of relevance to a story with a remote setting.

The virulence of epidemics may be exaggerated to increase the impact of a story. This was the case with early reporting of AIDS, which was treated as a new Black Death despite obvious differences in the way the disease is transmitted and develops. There was a genuine scare about millions dying of AIDS. The ethical issues concerning the way it was reported are:
- How much did anyone know at the time about how AIDS could be contracted?
- What justification was there for apportioning the blame (often in vindictive language) to gays?

The 'flesh-eating bug' scare of 1994 was almost entirely a media-produced story (Connor and Cohen, 1994) since the incidence of necrotising fasciitis had not increased significantly over previous years. As well as exaggeration, the media may get their facts wrong in the attempt

Read the following two accounts from the thalidomide tragedy and reflect on the feelings each arouses. Which is more effective at communicating information and getting you to react? What valid role do you think there is for sensationalism in relation to health care?

'The delivery team was upset to see that the baby was malformed. It had upper-limb abnormalities. In addition, there was a bowel atresia — the bowel had no opening.'

'One woman did not discover her child had no arms until she had taken him home and went to give him a bath. The hospital staff — and one can sympathize with them — had found it impossible to tell her.'

The *Sunday Times* Insight Team (1979) *Suffer the Children: The story of thalidomide*. London: André Deutsch.

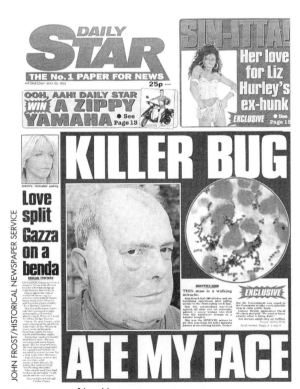

Coverage of healthcare issues can cause unwarranted panic

to sensationalise. Again, this happened with the early coverage of AIDS. Less excusably, since more is known, the *Sunday Times* said that *Streptococcus pyogenes*, responsible for necrotising fasciitis, also caused bubonic plague (Dixon, 1994).

A moralising context may also be given to healthcare reporting to increase the sensationalism. For example, herpes was presented in a moralist framework, as an 'epidemic' and 'incurable'; these terms were used to increase the impact and to stigmatise sexual promiscuity. Moralising in reporting is not restricted to news reporting: accounts of the failure of cosmetic surgery may also have a moral or disapproving slant. The focus tends to be on the personal experiences of particular women rather than surgical error, culpability, or how to prevent future occurrences.

Sensationalism and intrusion

Coverage of healthcare issues may invade the privacy of the people involved. Respecting the rights of patients/client informs all aspects of healthcare professionals' practice, but the media work to different codes. When television coverage of surgical operations began in the

1950s, the issue of the patients' privacy was quickly picked up on by healthcare professionals: 'the privacy of the surgical insult to a human body, even a consenting one, should be inviolable, and should never be made the basis of a Roman holiday for the titillation of the public's demand for thrills' (letter to the *BMJ*, March 8, 1958). The issue remains contentious in relation to programmes such as *Hospital Watch*, which trace the admission and treatment of real patients in real hospitals. Personal testimonies in programmes such as *Kilroy* also sometimes recount harrowing and deeply personal experiences of illness and surgery.

Sensationalist and irresponsible coverage of healthcare issues can cause unwarranted panic which may have health repercussions for readers and viewers. For example, scares about the contraceptive pill may cause women to stop taking it, with the result that referrals for terminations increase. People also worry about contracting illnesses they have seen covered in the media. As a result they may be reluctant to attend hospital if they fear they will pick up an infection. Stories of medical malpractice may also make people fear hospital admission.

'Whatever happens against custom we say is against Nature, yet there is nothing whatsoever which is not in harmony with her. May Nature's universal reason chase away that deluded ecstatic amazement which novelty brings to us.'
Montaigne, M. (1580) On a monster-child. Translated by Screech, M.A. (1991) *The Essays of Michel de Montaigne*. London: Allen Lane.

Look at some of the healthcare stories you have collected while you have been working on this unit. You might like to compare examples with others in your tutor/counsellor group. Do any of the stories sensationalise the issues? How do they achieve their effects? Why is there an inbuilt tendency for the media to be sensational?

Lies, damned lies . . .

There are lies, damned lies; and there are statistics. Statistics don't tell lies by themselves but they can be used by people who are telling lies to support the lie. The trick is to be clear what the statistic in each case is showing and to see how it relates to the things being said or written around it. Perhaps there is a lie in there. But the great thing about statistics is that they can reveal the lie just as easily as they can conceal it. For example, if the government claims that unemployment is lower than it was 15 years ago and uses a set of figures to support the claim, all you have to do is go back to the way the figures were counted 15 years ago and check that they are counting in the same way. They aren't, so it is easy to prove that the statement is a lie.

In the media, statistics are given more prominence the more dramatic they seem to be. In one newspaper report on the scare over the low dose contraceptive Pill in October 1995 (quoted below) the statistics are presented in order of importance. First they say that one-and-a-half million women are at risk — the larger the number of people affected, the more important the story. Then they say these women are 'twice as likely' to suffer thrombosis as women taking

other brands. But at this point we don't know the size of the risk. There are a further three paragraphs (not quoted here) before the size of the risk is revealed.

In this case, the choice of statistics probably goes back to the press release which sparked off the story. Media coverage of the Pill scare did not highlight the difference between non-Pill users and low-risk Pill users as this would call Pill use into question, which was not the object of the press release (see pages 114–115 for more on press releases). Information that the risk from the implicated Pills was much lower than the risk of thrombosis arising from pregnancy, childbirth and abortion was given little prominence and in some cases not mentioned. Yet this is important information. Some women may have stopped taking the Pill because they were scared by the story, and put themselves at greater risk through chancing an unwanted pregnancy.

Interpreting the evidence

As the volume of information grows, more statistics are used in reporting. This is because complex information can often best be presented statistically, for example in a graph or

'Row as women are warned of blood clot risk

'Women could be at risk from some brands of the Pill, experts warned last night. The million-and-a-half women taking seven low-dose varieties are twice as likely to develop blood clots as those who take other brands...

'A report states that 30 women in every 10,000 are at risk of developing thrombosis with low-dose brands of the Pill, compared to 15 in every 10,000 for other varieties. That is six times the number expected among young women who are not taking oral contraception.'

New scare over the Pill. *Daily Express*, October 20, 1995.

Women who take any oral contraceptive pill have four times the chance of developing thrombosis compared to women who do not take any. Is there necessarily a link? Think of the other factors that may influence the figures. For instance, women taking the Pill are sexually active; those who are not taking it may not be.

The guidelines for advising women about continuing to take the low-dose Pill said that it could be prescribed to women who were intolerant of other oral contraceptives and who accepted the increased risk. How would you feel about the risk yourself? How would you respond to a patient or client who asked you about it?

In retrospect, stories like the above often seem more alarmist than they need to be. Find out how this issue (or another one you know about from the recent past) is being reported now. To what extent are the reports more balanced and less alarmist after the passage of time? Why is this?

'If statistics are presented, how were they obtained? How confident can we be of them? Were they derived from a random sample or from a collection of anecdotes? Does the correlation suggest a causal relationship or is it merely a coincidence?...Do such figures measure what they purport to measure?'

Paulos, J.A. (1995) *A Mathematician Reads the Newspaper*. London: Penguin.

table. Part of being a good reader of the media is the ability to interpret statistics and to evaluate them critically – as one professor of mathematics says: 'Always be smart; seldom be certain' (Paulos, 1995).

Statistics may tell us whether there is a relationship or not between data, but they are not always conclusive. During the late 1980s, unemployment and house repossessions escalated. So did spending on bottled mineral water. We do not conclude that unemployed people or people whose homes have been repossessed are more likely to buy bottled mineral water than others. Nor that drinking mineral water makes you more likely to lose your job or home. We know from our own experience that these are unlikely consequences. But we can link the rise in unemployment with the rise in repossessions by looking at other evidence to help us draw these conclusions.

Knowing about a subject and its context makes it possible to judge whether there is likely to be a causal relationship between data. If readers or viewers do not know about the context, they tend to rely on the reporter's interpretation of the statistics unless there is something to make

them suspicious, such as political bias. A critical eye will often help to tell whether or not the inference drawn from statistics is reasonable.

Is it significant?

There are several methods for deciding whether a statistical result is 'significant', that is, whether it points to a real relationship or whether it could have been produced by chance. The formulae for testing significance can be quite complex. You may have used some in your work.

One study found that there was no significant increase in parasuicides following the depiction of a failed suicide attempt in an episode of *EastEnders* (Platt, 1987). Yet individual casualty departments noted a considerable increase. Discrepancies like this may sometimes be resolved by further research.

Researchers have to be careful that other factors do not distort their statistical findings. For instance, Schüklenk et al. (1995) claim that the transmission rate of AIDS from women to men is lower than reported because researchers have been misled by men who deny homosexual contact or intravenous drug use because of the stigma attached.

Researchers on the *Cook Report* (November 17, 1994; December 1, 1994) found that 50% of babies who died of sudden infant death syndrome (SIDS) had unusually high levels of antimony in their body tissues. Of these, 95% had definitely slept on mattresses that had PVC covers treated with a fire retardant containing antimony. There is no other significant source of antimony in the domestic environment.

From this information, would you conclude that the babies were poisoned by their mattresses?

Whether or not you believe a link exists, would you personally put your baby to sleep on a mattress you knew contained antimony?

Discuss with colleagues and/or others in your tutor/counsellor group:

- What criteria might be used to make an assessment of the risk in cases like these
- How to assess the statistical size of the risk when making decisions
- How you might balance the disruption to your lifestyle with the seriousness of the possible consequences of healthcare choices.

'The peasants say that a cold wind blows in late spring because the oaks are budding... But though I do not know what causes the cold winds to blow when the oak-buds unfold, I cannot agree with the peasants that unfolding of the oak-buds is the cause of the cold wind, for the force of the wind is beyond the influence of the buds. I see only a coincidence of occurrences such as happens with all the phenomena of life.'

Leo Tolstoy, *War and Peace*. Translated by Louise Maude and Aylmer Maude (1991). Oxford: Oxford Paperbacks.

Not in the news

The coverage of healthcare issues in the media does not reflect accurately the incidence of illness or healthcare provision in the community. The more sensational and newsworthy items get a lot of coverage, but the mundane, run-of-the-mill, unglamorous conditions that make up most people's experience of illness and use of healthcare services are under-represented. This is to some extent inevitable given that the media value their role as entertainers higher than their role as educators. An unproblematic operation, a non-life-threatening disease, a common injury is not thought interesting in its own right. It may occasionally find itself the subject of a feature or documentary, but generally only if some new treatment or controversy makes it topical for a while.

Unlike the rest of the media, professional journals cover the full range of medical conditions and healthcare issues, although the content of these journals may be skewed towards research funding — areas that are not funded may get less coverage — and/or advertising.

Patients on screen and in real life

A disproportionately large number of the patients featured in television documentaries and dramas are children. Relatively few are elderly people with chronic conditions, although they make up the majority of patients in reality. Television tends to glamorise; young, attractive patients with interesting or unusual conditions are more glamorous than elderly people with pressure sores and varicose ulcers. When elderly people with medical conditions are featured, it is often as the butt of jokes. Common, embarrassing or debilitating conditions such as incontinence, senile dementia and arthritis are used to characterise elderly people in comedies but are rarely afforded serious treatment.

One notable exception was Dennis Potter's drama *The Singing Detective*, which featured a depressive character with a painful skin condition (psoriasis). His condition was explored sensitively and honestly, including the shame and disgust he felt, the response of his family and others, and the pain and depression it caused him.

Health is attractive to the media because it affects everyone and is often emotive — two strong reasons for bringing health into the realm of entertainment (serious or otherwise). To what extent can the media inform and educate people about health as well as entertain them? What can be learned through empathy with characters and situations in a TV programme that portrays a health-related issue?

Some of the medical and healthcare topics covered in professional journals affect many people. Why do you think these topics do not receive coverage outside the professional press? How would you feel about giving patients/clients access to relevant articles in these journals? If you do not already do this, why not?

When the Queen Mother had a hip replacement operation in November 1995, her status as a newsworthy figure brought this routine operation into the limelight. All the national papers covered the operation. Because there was relatively little to say about the operation itself, coverage was extended by explaining what a hip replacement operation involves. For the thousands of people who have this operation every year, the coverage was probably a welcome recognition of their experience. They may have found the detailed descriptions and diagrams informative and reassuring.

There is more on ways of knowing and learning in the unit *Values and the Person: Ideas that influence health care*.

People with more 'interesting', high profile conditions such as cancer, AIDS and heart disease see quite a lot of media coverage of their experience. This can bring psychological and practical benefits. They may learn about new methods of treatment, or symptom relief. They will know that others have some knowledge of their condition and insight into their experience. Instead of the feelings of isolation which illness can create, they have a recognised place in the social experience. They may or may not like the way they are portrayed but at least they are given a voice and acknowledged. People whose condition is rarely or never represented may feel left out, undervalued and ignored, not specifically because there is no media coverage of varicose ulcers (or whatever) but because there is no public validation of their experience.

Feelings about illness

People who are ill are generally shown in one of two ways: valiantly battling against their condition, survivors at heart even if they will eventually succumb; or as victims who are to be pitied, helped and cared for by others.

This does not cover the wide range of responses people have to illness. Other aspects include disgust, shame, anger, resentment, hatred of their carers, fear, depression, boredom, mood swings and personality change. People who experience these may be afraid to talk about them. If they do, they may be put down or ignored by others who are not prepared for these responses because they do not fit in with the established pattern of representation of illness.

As part of your assessment for this unit, you might decide to conduct a quantitative survey of the types of illness represented, and the aspects of health care covered, in the materials you have collected while working on this book. For example, you could analyse whether the level of coverage you find corresponds to the real incidence of the conditions.

You can get *The Singing Detective* on video. Watch all or part of it, focusing on the way the central character's illness is treated. You might like to write a critique of this programme — or of some other fiction featuring central characters with a medical condition — as part of your assessment for the unit.

How are the conditions that affect the patients or clients you are working with at the moment discussed or represented in the media?

Talk to some of your patients or clients about the representation and find out whether they feel it is accurate. Is it a positive experience for them to see their condition represented or discussed?

If there is little or no media coverage, ask how they feel about being excluded.

Images of health and illness

Images of health and health care in the media help to form people's ideas of what it is to be healthy or ill. Media images of health conventionally show people who are young, slim, fairly attractive and who take exercise. They are likely to be shown in an active pose or situation, involved in social activity or dialogue. They do not have any obvious medical conditions or disabilities. This is an uncomplicated portrayal, but it is not at all comprehensive and does not relate directly to the diverse, complex ways in which each person perceives his/her state of health. Sometimes, a condition which may be well managed and does not interfere with general health may be shown in the media as an illness; for example, asthma, diabetes, impaired vision.

Portrayals of illness

There are many ways to look at the portrayal of illness in the media. Examples are:

- Associations and representations of different types of illness — acute and chronic illness, life-threatening and non-life-threatening illness
- Features of illness that are highlighted in programmes or characters
- The ill person as a social icon — patient, victim, survivor, for example

- The ill person's role in an article or programme
- 'Real' and fictional portrayals.

Portrayals of illness usually fit into set models or frameworks. For example, in a news story an ill or injured person may be shown as a helpless victim, pathetic sufferer, someone who has been wronged, a brave survivor, someone battling for survival or the passive object of medical intervention. In a magazine feature, a person triumphing over adversity to find new strength or to channel anger into constructive action are commonly shown as consequences of serious illness, for ill people and carers.

Other types of programmes or articles use different models. A situation comedy may make a mockery of illness and injury. The vulnerability of the patient in traction is a common icon, as is the dodgy heart which makes elderly people vulnerable to shocks or surprises. In these portrayals, the misery, pain and depression attendant on illness are absent. The condition becomes an identifying marker of the person and defines the person's role. In a medical documentary or *Hospital Watch*-type programme, the ill person's individual

During pregnancy, a healthy person may be subject to much medical attention, investigation and perhaps intervention. Pregnant women are no longer considered to be ill just by nature of their condition (though some may be ill as well as pregnant). Even so, visits to doctors and hospital clinics mean they may feel that they are treated as though they are ill.

Look at some images of pregnant women in magazines, on television, or in catalogues. Professional journals for midwives and other healthcare professionals may also contain a range of images. What positions and situations are the women shown in? Do they look like patients? Do they look healthy? Do you think these images will make pregnant women and people who care for them professionally view pregnancy as a state of health?

The social resonance and portrayal of TB, cancer and AIDs are discussed in:

Sontag, S. (1991) *Illness as Metaphor*. London: Penguin Books.

'...on the one hand, the press photograph is an object that has been worked on, chosen, composed, constructed, treated according to professional, aesthetic or ideological norms...; while on the other, this same photograph is not only perceived, received, it is *read*, connected more or less consciously by the public that consumes it to a traditional stock of signs.'

Barthes, R. (1982) The photographic message. In: Sontag, S. (ed) *A Roland Barthes Reader*. London: Vintage (reprinted 1993).

experience may be explored in a particular context, or it may be ignored completely, with the ill person shown as just an object of medical attention. In a programme or professional article about an operative technique, we may never see the patient as a whole person and never hear the person's voice. The patient is treated as a body.

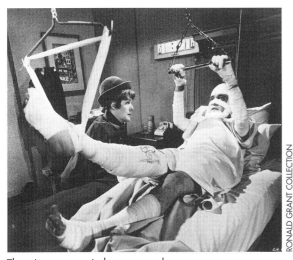

RONALD GRANT COLLECTION

There's a person in here somewhere

Some types of illness are rarely considered outside professional journals, or have very few modes of representation (see pages 68–69). Sometimes, portrayal of a group can be so negative that it is detrimental to real sufferers. For example, the widespread media coverage of HIV and AIDS may have led to AIDS sufferers being stigmatised and encountering real social problems, from victimisation to abuse. Some people may be afraid to admit to being HIV positive because the response of other people to media coverage of AIDS is unhelpful and ill-informed.

A starting point for your assessment for this unit might be to choose a form of the media and analyse its representation of health and illness. For example, you could look at situation comedies, TV soaps, magazine advertisements, professional journals or radio medical phone-ins.

Identify the ways in which illness and health are treated. See if you can work out:

- The shared understanding of health and illness they represent

- Any frameworks or models they are using for representations of ill people

- Whether they are representing people as social icons — patient, old person, dying person — or as individuals.

This could be a large-scale study, or something on which you spend quite a short time. You might decide to extend your study to other forms of media for the independent enquiry in the core degree unit, *Enquiring into Healthcare Practice*.

The unit *Health Promotion in Professional Practice* has a case study of the government's campaign to raise awareness of HIV/AIDS.

'To photograph is to appropriate the thing photographed. It means putting oneself into a certain relation to the world that feels like knowledge — and, therefore, like power.'

Sontag, S. (1977) *On Photography*. London: Penguin.

Disability and mental illness

Images of disability

News stories tend to present disability in four main ways:

- *'Tragic waste'* — as when the actor Christopher Reeve, who played the lead in the Superman films, became disabled after a riding accident. His career was built on his fitness and appearance, so media coverage focused on the waste of acting talent and physical ability
- *Accident or negligence* — the blinding of thousands of people in Bhopal in India, or the link between thalidomide and limb deformity. Big business and politics are the main players in the news arena: babies and distant Indian citizens are not. So this model tends to portray helpless victims and a culpable conglomerate
- *Courage and heroism* — there were many casualties of the Falklands War, but everyone has heard of at least one: Simon Weston, who suffered severe burning and facial disfigurement. He made his disfigurement public in the media, which reported the progress of reconstructive surgery and also normal events in his life, such as getting married
- *Hopeless case* — a few years ago, a policeman injured in a shooting lost the use of his legs. He appeared in the media, proclaiming his enthusiasm for the surgery and physiotherapy he was offered, saying he would never give up hope. Eventually, he became depressed and suicidal. The brief media coverage of this reversal was damning and unsympathetic: the hero had 'given in' to depression.

Features and documentaries are more thoughtful in their coverage of disability. They, too, tend to present it in four ways:

- *The medical approach* — concentrates on what can be done for the disabled in terms of cure or medical aids to help them live as normal a life as possible
- *The consumer approach* — addresses people with disabilities and their carers and aims to inform them about goods, services, benefits and rights. There is a strong self-help orientation
- *The look-after-yourself approach* — explains how to avoid particular types of disability (such as coronary problems) through healthy living. There is a subset on avoiding disability in the unborn child by giving up smoking and living healthily during pregnancy
- *The environmental approach* — emphasises the

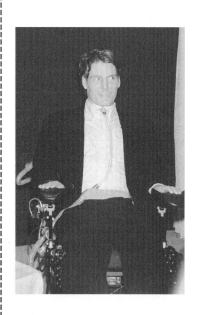
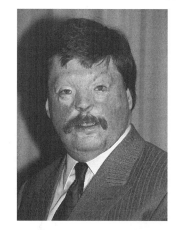
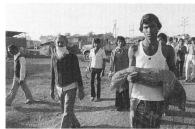
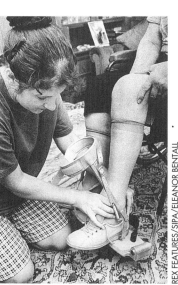

REX FEATURES/SIPA/ELEANOR BENTALL

What impression does each of these photographs convey about the person depicted? Look at their stance, their expression, their surroundings and work out how the photographer has manipulated the image to create the effect.

role of environmental and social factors in causing disability and the closing off of opportunities for disabled people.

Images of mental illness

Mental illness is most commonly shown as a threat to society. For example, a local newspaper might object to a hostel in the area for mentally ill people or a national news story might focus on how someone with mental illness has been released from care or custody and become a threat to society. The portrayal of mental illness in fictional contexts is rarely clinically accurate, perhaps reflecting a lack of both knowledge and interest on the part of the public. Media coverage of mental illness tends to stigmatise further an already disadvantaged and stigmatised group.

News stories of people released into 'care in the community' who then attack someone or kill themselves, deny any possibility of treating each psychiatric patient as an individual and assessing his or her own needs. They group all cases together as potentially dangerous. The public profile of people suffering from mental illness is also affected by the insensitive use of general and inaccurate terms such as 'mad', 'loony' and 'monster'. These may be applied to people with any type of mental illness (as in headlines such as 'Home for loonies to be sited near school'), to particular criminal cases ('Monster preys on lone women') or to people with no diagnosed mental condition ('Crazed youths wreck centre').

The respectable face of mental health in the media relates to stress, which is a major cause of mental illness and carries a certain degree of kudos — though the kudos is lost if the sufferer from stress becomes a sufferer from depression. Magazines for the professional classes carry articles on avoiding stress. Stress has become something of an executive accessory, even though it is actually people with little responsibility or control in their jobs, and the unemployed and poor, who suffer most from stress.

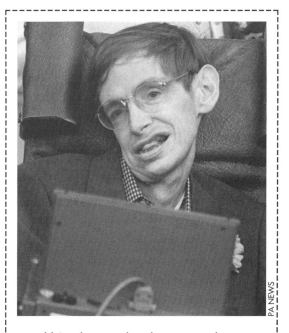

PA NEWS

Would Stephen Hawking have received so much media coverage if he had not been disabled? Has his exposure done anything to improve the lot of others suffering from motor neurone disease? Do you think it should have? Why do reports of his work mention his disability?

Shrinks was a drama series about psychiatry broadcast in early 1991. An ITC research paper examined audience response:

'The majority of viewers thought the series served to highlight public awareness of psychiatric problems and that it did so in a positive way... the vast majority thought that *Shrinks* helped to promote the view that it is acceptable to see a psychiatrist (72%) and to admit to having emotional, or psychiatric problems (71%). A smaller majority (56%) felt that the series encouraged a greater understanding of psychiatric problems and the difficulties such problems can cause sufferers and their families...'

Aldridge, J.S. (1991) *It's All in the Mind: Public opinion on the ITV series 'Shrinks'*. London: ITC Research Reference Paper.

If you know about mental health and illness from your practice, you could write a proposal for a radio or television programme, or a magazine or newspaper article on a mental health subject to increase awareness and understanding of a stigmatised social group.

Conclusion

This Section looked at the wide range of media forms that exist at the moment and how they present health care. But the media are always changing and developing, perhaps more quickly now than ever before. Your contact with the media in a professional capacity as well as your role as a private user will almost certainly bring you into contact with some of the new forms, such as specialised channels on cable and satellite and the use of the Internet to gain information.

The Section also raised issues about whether what the media present is true or reliable. As the role of computer technology in media production increases, questions of truth become increasingly complex. For example, a news agency may capture images from video or a satellite transmission on computer, digitally process them to cut out just the parts that are wanted and then print or distribute the picture to newspapers and broadcasters. The picture presented as the news photo has already been processed before the editorial team see it. There is no 'original' photograph, no negative, and maybe not even the original computer file against which to compare the pictures printed or broadcast.

New developments on the horizon will add to the number of media formats available to some people. It is impossible to tell now what effect they will have on the delivery of healthcare information and news, but in the short-term many of the more advanced (and expensive) forms will be available only to privileged sections of the community. The use of television for other functions — accessing library information, teleshopping and playing computer games — may also affect people's ways of viewing.

First reports of uprisings in out-of-the-way places are often now communicated over the Internet. Information from the USSR during its dissolution could not be stemmed by officials as it came to the West by e-mail. Chinese state authorities are so worried about information entering and leaving the country by e-mail and the Internet that they are planning to allow only one, state-controlled, Internet service-provider which would allow limited access to outside sources.

References

Bardo, S. (1990) Reading the slender body. In: Jacobs, M., Fox Keller, E. and Shuttleworth, S. (eds). *Body/Politics. Women and the discourses of science.* London: Routledge.

Curran, J. and Seaton, J. (1991) *Power Without Responsibility: The press and broadcasting in Britain.* London: Routledge (fourth edition).

Coiera, E. (1996) The Internet's challenge to healthcare provision. *British Medical Journal* 312: 3–4.

Connor, S. and Cohen, N. (1994) Not really a plague, but not just hype. *Independent*, May 29, 1994.

Dixon, B. (1994) A rampant non-epidemic. *British Medical Journal* 308: 1576–1577.

Franklin, B. and Murphy, D. (1991) *What News? The market, politics and the local press.* London: Routledge.

Hamilton, J.G.M. Letter to the editor. *British Medical Journal*, March 8, 1958, p577.

Karpf, A. (1988) *Doctoring the Media. The reporting of health and medicine.* London: Routledge.

Paulos, J.A. (1995) *A Mathematician Reads the Newspaper.* London: Penguin.

Platt, S. (1987) The aftermath of Angie's overdose: Is (soap) opera damaging to your health? *British Medical Journal* 294: 954–57.

Schüklenk, U., Mertz, D., Richter, J. (1995) The bioethics tabloids — How professional ethicists have fallen for the myth of tertiary transmitted heterosexual AIDS. *Health Care Analysis* 3(1): 27–36.

Smith, J. (1996) The value of nursing journals (editorial). *Journal of Advanced Nursing* 24(1): 1–2.

Winckler, M. (1984) Model women. In: Winckler, M. and Cole, L. (eds). *The Good Body: Asceticism in contemporary culture.* Newhaven and London: Yale University Press.

If you have access to the Internet, look at one of the on-line newspapers (eg www.the-times.co.uk).

Think about how you use a paper newspaper and how you use an on-line paper. What issues will the media have to address in the future, in relation to engaging their audience, if they move further in this direction?

Introduction

What people do with media messages determines the impact the media have and the influence they exert. This Section looks at how people respond to healthcare coverage in the media: whether they seek it out, take an interest in it, or ignore it completely, and what this says about the relationship between the media and their audiences?

People's use of the media can satisfy specific requirements. Subscribing to a professional journal may be a statement that the journal is useful and will be attended to closely, or it may be a career statement — many people buy professional journals for the jobs. Switching on the television to see what is on is, however, a much more casual engagement. But whenever people make a choice, even if it is just to leave on a programme they have found by chance, they are using the media to achieve a purpose. Except when a radio or television programme is left on for background noise, use of the media always means something. Information might be being given about things of which we have little or no direct experience, but where information about topics we know about is being given, there may be a conflict between our own interpretation of the experience (experienced meaning) and the meaning the media put on the event or issue (mediated meaning).

The wide range of media choice makes it possible for people to choose programmes, newspapers and magazines that are familiar and that generally reinforce rather than challenge their ideas and experiences too much. It is not too difficult to filter information and pay more attention to publications or programmes that endorse existing views and reject or ignore other material. Think about how you respond to programmes that put forward a political view contrary to your own. You may turn them off; you may dispute their statements; but you probably don't rethink your ideas in the light of them. Why are the media so unsuccessful at challenging people's ideas?

Think about the media choices you make. Build up a profile of:

- What you are using the media for — the purposes
- What your choices reflect about how you see yourself
- The extent to which the media challenges the way you think.

'Where experienced meanings are at odds with mediated meanings, a "negotiation" takes place in which both can be modified. But, of course, they can stay at odds, too, remaining "in contradiction". Second, mediated meanings are important in structuring the ways in which we see the world — even the world of experience.'

Hartley (1982) *Understanding News*. London: Methuen. (Reprinted 1988, Routledge, London.)

How people use the media

The type of attention people give to the media can be indicated along a continuum of reflection and active interpretation to passive reception. The type of medium determines the type of attention. For example, a newspaper or magazine can be read in any sequence: readers can pick out articles, give up on them or read them through again. Newspaper reading is selective; people rarely read a paper from cover to cover and if articles are not read by the end of the day they are usually not read at all. Magazines may have a longer shelf-life and professional journals may be kept indefinitely. On-line media give readers even more control over their choice of what to read: it is often possible even to choose whether or not to view pictures that accompany an article.

In general, people give closer, more focused attention to print than to broadcast media. In radio and television, the sequence is controlled by the broadcasters; at any moment the listener or viewer has less choice. Also, it is harder to get a sense of the content in advance — you cannot skim through a broadcast programme as you can a journal article. Furthermore, it is harder to review a broadcast programme critically, because there is not time, without a recording, to question the presentation or analyse the way, the programme works.

Programme scheduling aims to capture viewers for as long as possible. There are two common techniques, based on two models, of the way the scheduling of television programmes is done:
- *'Hammocking'* — a weak or potentially unpopular programme is sandwiched between two programmes that will attract viewers. The assumption is that people will sit through the dull programme to see the interesting one that follows
- *'Inheritance factor'* — popular programmes are broadcast early in the evening in the hope that people will not bother to switch channels when they have finished and that the viewers will 'inherit' the following programmes.

A 'uses and gratifications' theory (McQuail, 1987) suggests that audiences use the media to gratify their needs. Need affects both their selection and interpretation: people turn to a magazine article for information, or a television comedy for entertainment, and they interpret what they find in the light of their needs for gratification. These needs may be for:
- Information
- Entertainment
- Social interaction
- Maintaining or constructing personal identity.

Keep track for a few days of the situations in which you find yourself using print and broadcast media. Make brief notes of:
- What else you are doing at the time
- Whether you give your full attention to what you are reading, listening to or watching — use a scoring system such as 0-5.

At the end of the few days, analyse your own media use. Do you use the media mostly to get information, or mostly for entertainment? How do you use different types of media differently?

'Today the concept of literacy comprises many media. An enlightened policy on literacy must take into account the possibilities of all these media. Educational concerns must be extended to the whole of the media.'

Eco, U. (1995) The future of literacy. In: *Apocalypse Postponed*. London: HarperCollins.

Average reach (penetration of possible market) of TV channels, 1991	Daily %	Wkly %	Hrs:mins per wk
BBC1	65	91	9:07
BBC2	33	77	2:25
Any or all BBC	69	92	11:32
ITV	63	90	10:18
C4/S4C	34	77	2:12
Any commercial	67	92	12:30

BBC Annual Report and Accounts 1990/91.

Who uses what?

Statistics on media use are compiled from audience research (for broadcast media) and market research (for print media). The most important and influential figures are published by the:

- BARB (Broadcasters' Audience Research Board) — broadcast media
- ABC (Audit Bureau of Circulation) — print media
- BBC — publishes its own analysis of audience research annually.

Figures for viewing and listening are extrapolated from the reported use of a sample of the population. Circulation figures for printed media are more precise: the publishers can tell how many copies of their newspaper or magazine have been sold. But sales are not the same as readership. The viewing figures for a television programme relate to the number of people who (probably) saw the programme, but the circulation figures for a newspaper relate to the number of copies sold.

The way people interpret the messages they get from a programme or publication depends on many factors, including their own experiences, opinions, social status or class, prior level of knowledge and their level of interest in the topic.

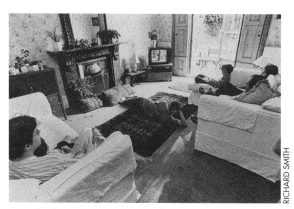

RICHARD SMITH

How do the media gratify people's needs?

Since social class is an important determinant of how people respond to messages, some audience and market research breaks down the viewing or circulation figures to give some idea of user profile. A common method for dividing people is by social group, as outlined below.

New technology is enabling the media to become increasingly personalised for individual users. This will offer an interesting challenge to the research bodies who track people's use of the media.

Research into audience and media consumption figures sometimes uses these categories for socio-economic groups:

A Higher managerial, administrative or professional

B Intermediate managerial, administrative or professional

C1 Supervisory or clerical, junior managerial, administrative or professional

C2 Skilled manual worker

D Semi-manual worker, unskilled manual worker

E State pensioner, widow (no other earner in household), casual or lower grade worker, unemployed

---

Circulation figures for national daily newspapers (average daily sales figures for October 1995):

Sun	5,055,746
Daily Mirror	2,522,501
Daily Mail	1,853,236
Daily Express	1,251,431
The Daily Telegraph	1,052,592
Daily Star	748,363
Times	675,032
Guardian	405,716
Financial Times	297,382
Independent	296,869
Total	14,158,868

Source: *Guardian*, November 18, 1995.

Reading and misreading

When reading, the individual's mind constructs meaning out of words, pictures, symbols, noises and other external stimuli. People have a range of highly intelligent strategies for bringing meaning to language and they are just as involved in this constructivist enterprise as the people who produced the text, programme or other utterance: 'Language makes sense — it is meaningful — when meaning can be brought to it. In fact, I would define *meaning* as "the relevance that can be imposed on an utterance"... In my view, reading is not a matter of decoding letters to sound but of bringing meaning to print' (Smith, 1983).

Television uses a code and assumes — rightly or wrongly — that most viewers can be expected to understand and interpret it correctly. Broadcasters present a message using their own framework of cultural reference: 'This framework which we could call ideology... constitutes a system of assumptions and expectations which interacts with the message and determines the selection of codes with which to read it' (Eco, 1980). According to Eco, television makes use of a three-part code: iconic, linguistic and sound-based (see panel below). If viewers recognise and use the information needed to decode the message, they can decode it as the producer intended, although producers do not necessarily expect viewers to share the same meanings. There are often 'flags' to help decode images and text. For example, if a reporter in a health programme says we should eat four pieces of fruit a day, the context tells us that we should do this to remain healthy, not to make agriculture economically viable.

What happens when a programme is not interpreted within the range of interpretations that the producer envisaged? Eco calls this 'aberrant decoding'. Is the message viewers take away really 'aberrant' (that is, wrong) or does it have its own validity? One study of how viewers understood a *Nationwide* broadcast differently demonstrated how the 'meaning' of a television programme is contingent upon the viewers' own ideologies and sociological profiles (Morley, 1980).

At one time, audience research measured whether viewers had understood and accepted the message the producer intended (the 'preferred reading'). A more sophisticated model asks instead what people do with the media messages they receive. It doesn't matter what the producer intended, the 'audience... "created" the media message in response to their own needs

Television codes

The iconic code has four subcodes:

- Iconological — some images have acquired particular connotations by tradition, for example, a smiling child running towards an old person connotes grandparent and grandchild
- Aesthetic — accepted ideas of beauty bestow meaning on images according to convention
- Erotic — accepted ideas of what is sexually attractive bestow meaning on images, again according to convention
- Montage — meaning comes from the sequence or juxtaposition of images.

The linguistic code includes sub-codes of specialist jargon and stylistic conventions. Style can connote social class, artistic attitude, emotional resonance. Viewers can tell whether something is ironic by judging whether it offends an accepted code deliberately or accidentally.

The sound-based code helps viewers to interpret music and sound effects. There is an emotional code, such as music associated with menace. Different types of music are linked with different ideologies. There are also types and sequences of sound that have a conventional value, for example, a drum roll followed by silence.

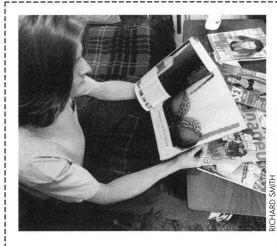

RICHARD SMITH

What information do you need to be able to decode this advertisement correctly? If you did not have this information, how do you think you would interpret the picture? What validity would an 'alternative' or 'aberrant' decoding have?

and their predisposition which shaped their interpretations' (Karpf, 1988). A final model combines elements of both: viewers and programme-makers both produce messages. Some viewers find the preferred reading, while others make their own message or disagree with the preferred reading. The general consensus now seems to be that 'meaning is the product of particular interpretative conventions (variously commonplace or esoteric) being applied to textual imagery and language' (Richardson and Corner, 1986).

Reading the press

The account given in different newspapers of the same event is often quite different. On January 11, 1996, the BMA issued a statement criticising the lack of emergency hospital beds and warning that it could have serious consequences.

The *Daily Express* headed its coverage by photographs of the 'opponents', health minister Stephen Dorrell and head of the BMA, Dr Sandy Macara, on opposite sides of the headline: 'Condition critical as bed crisis puts lives in danger'. Along the top of the page ran the line: 'Accident victims kept on stretchers in hard-pressed hospitals'. At the foot of the page there

was a photograph of Geoffrey Cranswick, who had had a heart attack, could not be found a bed and died after being air-lifted to another hospital. The coverage focused on conflict between the doctors and the government and on the human interest aspect of the fate of patients. This fits into a standard model of reporting: the article does not analyse the aims of the two parties and leaves it to readers to put their own interpretation on the model.

The *Independent* flagged its coverage of the issue as 'Analysis'. It included a catalogue of bed shortages in different hospitals. The title of the main article is: 'Doctors call for retreat on internal market' and the banner across the top of the article read: 'Hospital crisis: BMA urges Government to reconsider strategy as problems deepen'. The article did not mention patients waiting on trolleys, or the death of Geoffrey Cranswick. Instead, it tried to work out why there was a crisis in emergency admissions and cited the rise in admissions as a main cause. It accounted for this by outlining changes in patient and GP behaviour. The coverage treated both doctors and ministers as partners in policy-making, seeking a solution rather than setting up opposition.

Why do you think coverage in the *Independent* showed more interest in the healthcare policy which led to the beds crisis than its results in human terms? Why did the *Daily Express* cover the consequences for patients and not try to analyse the situation at all?

In a survey conducted in 1986, nurses claimed that the *Guardian* gave the fairest and most accurate reporting of health care and nursing issues, and the *Sun* was among the worst.

Nursing Times (1987) Vox pop. Media casualty? *Nursing Times* 83(4): 22.

Items on healthcare crop up frequently in the press and on television. Look out for a topic over the next few days, and compare the treatment given to it by different newspapers, radio and television.

If you study several newspapers, can you find consistent differences between the coverage in the broadsheets and the tabloids?

To what extent do the programmes and publications rely on the sort of extended code that comes from being familiar with the context? What sense would someone outside the context make of them?

Disjunctive reporting

Editors and programme-makers usually maintain some degree of consistency in the type of coverage but there can also be a lot of disjunction, particularly in print media. Articles are likely to be consistent within themselves, but there may be contradictions across the spread of a newspaper or magazine, so that readers are responsible for making their own interpretation (or ignoring the disjunction).

Advertising sometimes leads to disjunctions. For example, the editorial copy in a magazine may promote a healthy diet, while the advertisements it carries push unhealthy foods and diet 'remedies' that are supposed to cure the ills caused by the junk food. Occasionally, magazines respond to reader pressure to drop advertising for a certain product or type of product.

Disjunction has a function that may or may not be intended, but it is valuable anyway — it encourages more critical reading of the content and reflection on the points of contact between issues not previously thought about together.

Common types of disjunction in editorial pages are:
- Using very thin models on the fashion pages,

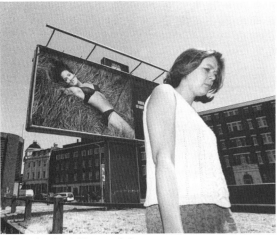

RICHARD SMITH

What do *I* look like in a bikini?

but advising sensible weight control, sensible diet and warning of the dangers of anorexia. Very thin models in magazines and on the cat-walks have been blamed for the increase in eating disorders among young women
- Using titillating images of women but reporting on sexual violence, which may be encouraged by the view of women such images give
- Including recipes for foods high in sugar and saturated fat, but running articles on eating a healthy diet.

'Disjunctive: tending to separate...indicating an alternative or opposition'

Chambers Dictionary (1994). Edinburgh: Chambers Harrap Publishers Ltd.

Disjunctive reporting may arise because there is genuine disagreement or lack of clarity about issues. This is especially true if the issues have a moral dimension, as with reports about patients in persistent vegetative states (PVS). The unit *Values and the Person: Ideas that influence health care* explores different ways of thinking about difficult issues.

- Using photographs that uphold conventional notions of beauty while running copy that rejects such notions as chauvinistic, oppressive or limiting

There may also be disjunction between articles. For instance, a compassionate article on how a woman loves her disabled child might be next to a piece on pre-natal testing which enables women to abort a fetus if the child will be born with serious disabilities. There may be dissonance or disjunction within an article. The extract from *Chat* magazine printed below starts by applauding the woman's figure, even though it goes on to reveal that she is slim because she has an eating disorder. Writing like this is not a helpful way to address women who may be concerned about their diet and weight.

Does it matter?

In some ways disjunction is a benefit. It is not necessary for a magazine to have a fixed policy on every issue, and showing the complexity of different perspectives is often constructive and liberating. But for some issues, the adverse implications for health may argue for a stronger editorial line. For instance, is it right to use ultra-thin models when this may be pyschologically and physically damaging to the kinds of readers the magazine is aiming to attract?

One area in which disjunction may be particularly damaging is in the 'advertorial' or promotional editorial now run by many magazines as a source of advertising revenue. Here, often unhealthy products are apparently endorsed and promoted by the magazine. Is this an abuse of influence?

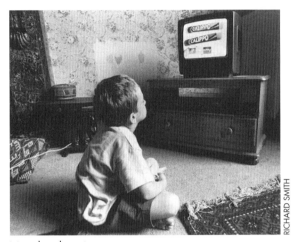

Naughty, but nice

'Most women would envy Diane Hague's trim figure. But her good looks hide a tortured past. First anorexic — her weight dropped from 8 stone to 5 stone — then suffering from bulimia, her obsession with food has cost her two marriages and a promising business, and left her with heavy debts and a lifetime of lies.'
Food junkies. *Chat*, February 6, 1988.

The unit *Professional Relationships: Influences on health care* uses the term 'cognitive dissonance'. It means that people can sometimes be aware of contradictory impulses or imperatives without feeling they have to reconcile them. For example, although people are aware of the risks of smoking, they may occasionally feel that the pleasure they (or a patient/client) gets from smoking outweighs the risks in their case.

Ask others in your tutor/counsellor group what they think about the disjunction found in many magazines.

Do they feel that people notice and draw their own conclusions, or do they generally not notice the disjunction at all?

Is it patronising to suggest that people will be confused by the conflicting messages, or is a pluralistic approach positively beneficial?

Do they want editors to take a stronger line on some healthcare issues?

Seeking out healthcare coverage

Much science reporting in newspapers and general interest magazines is related to medicine and health. Health care features in news, documentaries, dramas, films and discussion programmes. Partly this is because health and illness are universal experiences, like love and death. But there may be other reasons why people seek out information on health at particular times. Karpf (1988) has shown that healthcare coverage waxes and wanes according to social factors. When people feel less in control of other aspects of their lives — during recession and war, for example — they show more interest in taking charge of their physical and mental well-being, devoting time and attention to health care.

People may look for specific items of healthcare coverage for many reasons:
- Information about a condition or aspect of health — they will follow media coverage if it appears at the right time, but are more likely to seek advice directly from a reference book or a healthcare professional
- Advice on healthy living and preventive measures for themselves or for people they care for
- Information about conditions they are afraid

they may develop, or about healthcare settings (for reassurance or so that they are not afraid of the unknown)
- Voyeurism — they want to see the experiences of others, particularly unpleasant experiences
- They want to see their own conditions or problems covered in the media to give a context and validity to their experiences.

Information and misinformation
Neuberger (1994) points out the value of an informed and informative media in relation to health and medicine: 'Proper information might well lead people to use the services of the NHS more discriminatingly and more efficiently'. She identifies two categories of information which should be available in an open society:
- Information which allows individuals and organisations (patients/clients and health service-providers) to make choices
- Information which allows them to participate fully in the democratic community and public debate over health care.

The media are an important source of information, but do people understand the information they see? Media research suggests

---

'The public like to know... what men die of — and women, too.'

Lord Beaverbrook, quoted in: Curran, J. and Seaton, J. (1991) *Power without Responsibility. The press and broadcasting in Britain.* London: Routledge (fourth edition), p55.

Look at a copy of Holland, W.W. (1991) *The European Atlas of Avoidable Death.* Oxford: Oxford University Press (second edition). You should be able to find a copy in your library; if not, ask for it to be ordered. If people had access to this information on a daily basis, would it make any difference to them, or to your own practice?

The early media campaign to stop the spread of HIV caused confusion rather than giving people information on which to base choices about their behaviour:

'Editorial and marketing concerns about "offending" the readers or viewers often intervene. For example, the *Guardian* followed the practice of not using the term "anal intercourse" for a number of years.'

Miller, D., Kitzinger, J., Williams, K. et al. (1992) Message misunderstood. *Times Higher Education Supplement*, July 3, 1992.

that it is easy for a non-expert to misconstrue information given in good faith. A study of viewers' understanding of the causes of cancer after watching a programme on cancer revealed that many of them misunderstood or misremembered the message (Karpf, 1988). Many people quoted as carcinogenic substances which the programme had specifically said did not cause cancer. Because they heard them mentioned in the context of causes of cancer, they assumed they caused cancer. A study of what people remembered from and believed of media coverage of AIDS found that they were ready to believe items about AIDS being endemic in African countries, did not distinguish between different parts of the continent and were less critical of how the media presented AIDS in Africa than they were of how the media presented AIDS in the UK (Miller et al., 1992).

Inevitably, there will be imprecision in reporting complex healthcare issues. Some information is just wrong, as when the *Sunday Times* reported that necrotising fasciitis was caused by the same bacterium as bubonic plague (Dixon, 1994). It may seem that the way to make information easily digestible so that the possibility of misunderstanding is reduced is to present it in as simple a form as possible. But over-simplification can lead to its own problems. In 1995, Leah Betts died after taking Ecstasy (see page 31). The media coverage that followed condemned ecstasy as the culprit, but it seems likely that drinking an excessive amount of water afterwards probably contributed to her death.

'An analysis of media coverage of child abuse in 1991 found that 71% of press coverage and 83% of television news coverage was case-based. Only 9% was on how to intervene in cases of suspected abuse. The researchers argued that the media are missing opportunities to inform people about child abuse and help prevent it. When prevention is mentioned, it tends to use unhelpful but attention-grabbing words like "monster" and "child molester".'

Kitzinger, J. and Skidmore, P. (1995) Playing safe: Media coverage of child sexual abuse prevention strategies. *Child Abuse Review* 4 (1): 47-56.

'A question mark hung over Leah's death. Was it a direct reaction to the ecstasy tablet that killed her, or drinking gallons of water in the false belief that this is an antidote to the drug? If her story had been pushed in less simple terms, to include her way of death, perhaps it would have prevented Helen Cousins falling into a coma from drinking seven litres of water after taking ecstasy two months later... And if Leah Betts had been keen to take her knowledge of the danger of reacting to ecstasy by overdrinking water into young people's lives, would the tabloids and prime-time news programmes that splashed her face around as part of the "war against drugs" have helped to get this more pragmatic message out?'

Walter, N. (1996) Dead women who suit the news agenda. *Guardian*, January 18, 1996.

Social impact

Some media material aims to have a particular impact on society. Examples are propaganda and advertising. Other types of programme and publication may affect behaviour just as directly. On October 13, 1980, *Panorama* broadcast a programme on the methods used to determine whether a person was dead. It concluded that British tests for brain death were not sufficiently reliable to form the basis of a decision to transplant organs from a corpse. Both the programme itself and the *Radio Times* cited examples of people who had been pronounced dead but turned out to be alive after all. Remarks such as 'the results suggest that two people in every hundred are being labelled dead when they could make a full recovery' caused a dramatic reduction in the number of organs offered for transplant: patients in need of transplant organs died while waiting for an organ to become available.

A health promotion campaign may make deliberate use of many types of media, but still not be as effective as a 'scare' story like the *Panorama* investigation. The government's drive to reduce the risk of AIDS in the population, starting in 1985, used television, newspaper and magazine advertising, posters and leaflets to try to reach as many people as possible. But although understanding about AIDS increased as a result of the campaign, behaviour probably did not change. People outside the gay community were no more likely to use condoms after seeing broadcasts about the risk of AIDS than they had been before (Wober, 1987).

The variable impact of the *Panorama* programme and the AIDS campaign poses the question why some programmes are more persuasive than others. One reason may be that health promotion films tell people what to do in order to avoid or gain something — avoid fats and sugars to reduce your risk of heart disease; take exercise to improve your health. On the whole, people object to being told what to do, particularly by the government. Documentary broadcasts provide people with information on which they could base their own judgements about how they should act. It is a more empowering form.

Soap – cleaning up its act?

For many people, television soaps are a source of enjoyment and relaxation. They are also a source of information about drug abuse, prenatal testing, dealing with disease, depression,

---

There is more on the failures and successes of health promotion campaigns in the unit *Health Promotion in Professional Practice*.

Watch an episode of a soap critically. Look out for the lifestyle and habits of the characters. How much do they drink? What do they eat? Do they take exercise? Do they get themselves into situations that threaten their health? If any of the characters are ill, injured or pregnant, do they behave appropriately? If not, is there any direct criticism of their behaviour?

If you want to make a detailed critique of one or more episodes of a soap, make a video recording and write up your account of the presentation of lifestyle and health issues. You may be able to use this as part of your assessment for the unit. A more comprehensive study could form the basis of your enquiry-based project in the core unit, *Enquiring into Healthcare Practice*.

Look at this advertisement. Is it trying to encourage you to change your behaviour? Is it likely to work?

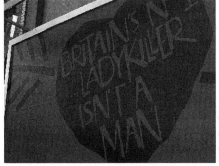

MICHAEL MELIA

A poster campaign gets to the heart of the matter. Beneath the image on the poster are the words: 'Heart-related illness kills 1 in 4 women. Help us fight it.'

If you want to experience at first hand the difficulty of getting people to change their behaviour, design a health promotion advertisement or poster yourself and try it out on some friends.

domestic violence, eating disorders and abortion. In 1995, *Neighbours* included a catalogue of health issues, including family mental illness, depression, bereavement, alcoholism, and bulimia. Two pregnancies were followed to term and involved a threatened miscarriage, high blood pressure, pre-eclampsia and Caesarean delivery. Soap producers consult healthcare professionals to get their facts right and to anticipate the effects of highlighting a particular issue. Sound medical advice is generally given in the storyline, but the soaps may also offer consolation, recognition and validation of people's feelings. When *Brookside* included a story in which a character had a Down's syndrome baby, viewers' letters ranged from criticism of the way it was handled to expressions of gratitude from people who recognised their own situation and were encouraged and comforted to see it covered.

The presentation of issues such as these often has moral overtones. One of the storylines in *Neighbours* centred on a group of teenagers who liked to race their cars recklessly. Eventually, one was killed when one of the cars crashed. Some of the 'good' characters had been involved, but had been shown to feel uneasy about participating, and had withdrawn from the final, fatal race. Several further episodes explored the legal consequences and the suffering and learning processes of the surviving participants.

Specific incidents in soaps can affect people's behaviour. When the *EastEnders* character Angie took an overdose but did not die in an episode broadcast on February 27, 1986, there was criticism from healthcare professionals, who reported a rise in parasuicides (Platt, 1987).

'Although mass hysteria and "copycat" behaviour are well-known, commonsense suggests that viewing a suicide attempt would have a discouraging effect. The BBC can hardly be blamed for not knowing in advance which tendency the programme would have. It is not reasonable to expect the BBC to desist from including in their programme stories with medical connotations.'
Fowler, B P. (1986) Emotional crises imitating television. *Lancet* 2 (8509): 750.

The healthcare consumer

The change towards a market economy and mentality within the NHS means that the end users of the service — patients, clients, healthy members of society — have taken on the role of consumers. This isn't just a change in terminology. People have begun to act as consumers, demanding consumer rights in the arena of health care and challenging the authority of doctors and other healthcare professionals. They have begun to look around at the options, including private health care and complementary therapies, and to demand a choice. You have probably noticed changes in your own area of practice in the ways people now interact with the health service and with healthcare professionals.

The media are playing an important part in this change of attitude and approach. People see media coverage of legal cases and complaints against service-providers, advertisements for healthcare products and services, and an increasing amount of information about health care. All of these combine to promote the role of consumerism and to make people increasingly sophisticated consumers (although not all the information people glean from the media is useful or properly understood: see pages 88–89).

Opening up the market

Most people want to use the NHS for their health care. Although independent health care is growing quickly, it is too expensive to be a real option for most of the population. This means that they do not have the usual consumer privilege of choice — of being able to take their business elsewhere if they are not satisfied. The new structure of providers and purchasers gives consumer power to purchasers, such as GPs, but not to the final consumers, the patients. This is an unusual structure in a market economy. For the end user, there is still a monopoly, but for the intermediate purchasers there is a free market with competition. Consumer panels for the public may provide information but have little authority.

Advertising for healthcare products and services and media-based health promotion campaigns encourage people to play a part both in looking after their health and in directing their treatment when they are ill. Self-diagnosis is encouraged by media content such as:
* Advertising for healthcare products and remedies
* 'Doctor' problem pages, columns and phone-ins
* Programmes and articles about particular conditions

'Patients have become more aware of their rights as consumers of health care; as a group they are more demanding. If they are not satisfied with the care they receive [from their GP], they self-refer to accident and emergency.'

Hunt, L. BMA urges rethink 'on internal market'. *Independent*, January 12, 1996, p4.

If you have access to the World Wide Web, consult the 'Web doctor' (http//www.telemedical.com).

This allows you to describe symptoms and get a diagnosis.

Do you think this service is useful? Or dangerous? How do you think it affects people's attitudes to health care and healthcare professionals?

Think of an example from your practice of someone coming to you with information gleaned from the media and suggesting a course of treatment or some other action on the basis of it. Perhaps the choice of drugs was queried or the diagnosis, or the question of using a complementary therapy was raised.

How did you feel about this person taking more control of his/her treatment? Did you discuss how the media had represented the treatment in the light of your experience as a healthcare professional? How would your understanding of the media inform this sort of discussion? You might like to note down your thoughts in your learning journal and discuss them with others in your tutor/counsellor group.

The unit *Complementary Therapies and Health Care Practice* contains more background information on the way these therapies have become more popular and available in the UK.

- Recorded message phone lines on health-related topics, advertised in the media
- News coverage of outbreaks of illness.

People are now being encouraged to consult their pharmacist rather than go to the doctor as a first line of inquiry for minor complaints. Remedies are available over the counter for a wider range of illnesses now that many drugs have been removed from prescription-only status and homoeopathic and other complementary remedies have also entered the consumer market. As a pharmacist works in a shop and sells remedies, patients are therefore being encouraged to see themselves as consumers.

Legal action against hospital trusts and individual healthcare professionals has now increased to the point where the media often lead on the legal rather than the health issues, as happened when the *Independent* covered the confusion of amniocentesis results which led a woman to abort her healthy baby (Cooper, 1985). As healthcare consumers, some people are following the commercial and industrial lead: if not satisfied, sue. As healthcare professionals take greater responsibility for clinical aspects of care, they may become more involved in legal actions.

Nowadays, people have more opportunity than ever to voice their concerns about treatment they have received. These complaints might relate to clinical treatment. They could also be about the ways in which complaints and/or their treatment have been dealt with by staff. Many believe that complaints are not taken seriously by trusts or acted upon. Of course it is always possible that a trust might choose to do little about a complaint made.

However, in my experience trusts take complaints very seriously. Complaints can be quite complex and often they take time to investigate, but by and large each complaint, at our trust at least, is carefully investigated. There is a complaints working group which monitors all complaints and makes recommendations for improving practice. Very often the nature of the complaint is so complex that the trust finds itself doing the work of preparing a case for litigation. This is becoming increasingly the case as people seek recompense for what they perceive to be bad service.

Cathy Hull, Non-Executive Director, Complaints Convener, Medway NHS Acute Trust.

'People used to feel warmly towards their local hospital. They would become involved in fund-raising for equipment, and campaign for it. As hospitals have become trusts people are seeing them more and more as businesses. Highly paid executives are seen as a drain on resources and are resented by the community. In the "us and them" polarisation of commerce, hospitals are now part of "them" and no longer of "us", the consumers.'

Penny, hospital administrator

Do you agree with the hospital administrator's assessment of people's change in attitude to their local hospital? (see above). Has it been obvious in your area of practice? What other ways are there in which becoming a consumer affects how people view the healthcare services they use and depend upon?

Do you think the increase in legal action against trusts is allied with their business-like image? Or would it have happened anyway as consumers became more aware and informed?

Impact on policy

Media coverage may have an impact on healthcare policy and practice. It can do this by:

- Putting an item up for public debate or raising the profile of an issue
- Mobilising public opinion or initiating public action
- Reflecting public concerns and putting pressure on policy-makers and government.

Three case studies

1. In January 1996, media coverage of the prison service's practice of shackling pregnant and labouring women during hospital visits built on campaigners' battles for reform and led to a reversal of Home Office policy. Individual midwives and other healthcare professionals had been working for a long time to get the practice changed and their efforts may have had a cumulative effect. But it was only after a prisoner's friend smuggled a video camera into a hospital and filmed the practice, then released the tape to the media, that action was taken. Both the press and broadcast media covered the practice extensively and the Home Office changed its policy within a few days.

2. The *Horizon* broadcast 'A time to be born' (January 1975) criticised the practice of routine induction for reasons of convenience rather than because it was medically necessary. The programme was based on articles in the *Sunday Times* and *Lancet*. It was slated in the *British Medical Journal* and raised questions in the House of Commons. But it brought about widespread criticism of the policy on induction and prompted a change in practice, allowing the voice of the mother to be heard and heeded.

3. When Cambridgeshire Health Authority refused to treat Jaymee Bowen for leukaemia, her father took the health authority to court. The media coverage of the case focused on the issue of the funding of expensive treatment with a low chance of success. The common perception was that the health authority had refused to treat Jaymee because the treatment would be expensive and she was unlikely to survive. The health authority maintained that it was a clinical decision based on weighing up the suffering she would endure against the chance of recovery.

Funding and resources

By making some issues high profile, media coverage affects the status of these issues. This in turn can affect allocation of resources for treatment and research: 'individual papers or

'Some urgent questions for the Ministry of Defence in London and the Department of Defense in Washington:

'If there is no such thing as Gulf War Syndrome, why are so many formerly healthy soldiers now in wheelchairs?

'If there is no such thing as Gulf War Syndrome, why are the wives of so many Gulf veterans sick?

'If there is no such thing as Gulf War Syndrome, why are so many parents with no history of genetic problems producing deformed and damaged babies?

'If none of the above is connected with the inoculations and pills issued to Desert Storm troops, why are so many veterans discovering that their medical records have gone missing?

'Why were some units warned not to conceive children for at least a year after taking the drugs?

'...If the Ministry of Defence has nothing to hide, why did the parliamentary committee trying to find answers to the above believe it had been misled?'

Miller, R. (1996) Children of the storm. *The Sunday Times* magazine, January 14, 1996.

Following extensive media coverage, partly prompted by pressure from victims and their families, on January 30, 1996, the government instigated an inquiry into whether there is such a thing as Gulf War Syndrome. This was a reversal of the government's earlier claim that there was no evidence of a syndrome and no need for an investigation.

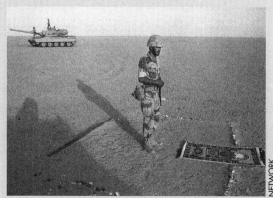

A battle for the truth

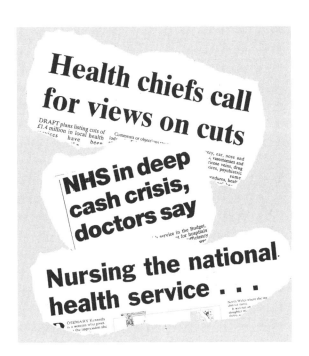

programs too often sensationalize and overplay stories, exaggerating risks and scaring the public... That, critics say, produces governmental responses — such as requiring removal of asbestos in schools or lead paint in homes — that may go much farther than scientifically justified, diverting money that might be better used to extend

prenatal care or vaccinate more children' (Otten, 1992).

One very particular way in which the media can focus attention on an issue is by crusading on behalf of a single sufferer, often a child. When *That's Life* ran an appeal on behalf of Ben Hardwick, suffering from biliary atresia, a liver donor was found and Ben had a transplant. Although Ben later died, the campaign had a lasting effect: 'We've battled and battled away to bring the problem of finding child donors to the attention of doctors and patients for three years. The story of Ben managed to do more in just one week. Kidney transplants rose by 40 per cent after Ben's story... The programme led to a House of Commons debate ... on how to increase the number of donors' (Karpf, 1988). But the health authority could not afford to run the intensive care room the appeal intended to provide. It is not uncommon for donations to provide equipment which is too expensive to use.

'Media campaigns such as *That's Life* intervene to affect NHS priorities, orienting them almost inevitably towards high-technology medicine. Their intervention isn't necessarily based on any measured consideration of competing needs, but more often determined by the cuteness of the patient.'

Karpf, A. (1988) *Doctoring the Media. The reporting of health and medicine.* London: Routledge.

What can be done to correct this? You might like to discuss the effect of media campaigns with others in your tutor/counsellor group, who may have their own direct experiences of the results of such campaigns.

Why did the media choose to fight the Home Office policy on women prisoners? You may be able to think of similar examples. The reasons may have something to do with their sensitivity to societal norms — how society would be likely to react to images of pregnant women in chains.

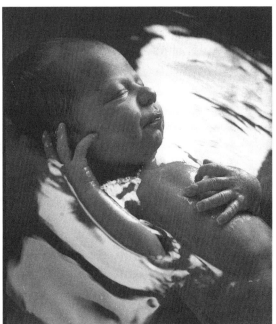

JON WALTER

A single case can help highlight an issue effectively

Images of the NHS

The dominant media view of the NHS is as a service beset by cutbacks, staff shortages and long waiting lists, increasingly subject to legal attacks by patients and weighed down by bureaucracy. It is a grim picture. Is this really what people believe? To what extent is it an image created by the media for its dramatic impact? What is the truth?

If you listen to people talking in the street, on the bus or with friends, you will probably hear a combination of damning tales and accolades. People seem to be able to hold contradictory attitudes about the NHS at the same time. It is not easy to find out exactly what they think. Results from some surveys into public attitudes are shown in the box below. The authors of the article presenting the results comment that: 'Subtle changes in media coverage contributed to displacing anxiety about the NHS from its position in the agenda of public consciousness. This may account for the fall in numbers of those dissatisfied with the running of the NHS between August and November 1991 [from 25.2% to 17.6%]. An apparent fall in dissatisfaction with the way the NHS runs must, however, be carefully interpreted. There is an inherent ambiguity in the question on satisfaction with the NHS. It elicits some combination of political views and personal experience, together with many other factors. Most importantly, perhaps changes in public opinion may be seen to reflect the effectiveness of management of news by the various interest groups' (Judge et al., 1992).

Frameworks of reporting

On pages 34–35, four models of healthcare reporting are outlined; the

- *Medical model* — focuses on high-tech medical intervention, miracle cures and the skill of doctors and surgeons
- *Consumer model* — focuses on the patients and their experiences
- *'Help-yourself' model* — makes individuals largely responsible for their own health
- *Environmental model* — acknowledges the importance of social and political factors in determining health.

Although the medical model has implications for the representation of the NHS, discoveries and breakthroughs are generally related to research institutes or individuals and successful operations are credited to the surgeons rather than the hospital teams and the NHS as a whole.

Changing attitudes to the NHS in the 1980s are shown in the results of two surveys carried out in 1990:

	1990	1983
Satisfied (very or quite)	37	55
Neither	15	20
Dissatisfied (very or quite)	47	25

	1990	1985
Positive	75	77
Neither	8	12
Negative	12	10
Don't know	5	1

Quoted in: Judge, K., Solomon, M., Miller, D. et al. (1992) Public opinion, the NHS and the media: changing patterns and perspectives. *British Medical Journal* 304: 893.

Do you think that most people's perceptions of the health service are based on simplistic concepts about a complex set of debates into priorities, cost-effectiveness, service levels, professional responsibilities, and so on.

If you are interested in this question of public perception, you could conduct a survey of your own into attitudes towards the NHS. You will need to decide what sort of survey to conduct and design an appropriate methodology. The core unit, *Enquiring into Healthcare Practice*, describes a range of enquiry methods and guides you through the process of conducting research.

If you don't want to do a survey, a few questions to friends and relatives may give you some insights into how people view the NHS and how important the media are in forming those views.

The consumer model, which perhaps has most relevance for the NHS, is most often used for negative portrayals — patients' rights violated or compromised, negligence, waiting lists and *The Patient's Charter*. The 'help-yourself' model encourages the view that people can help themselves to health, with or without the NHS. The environmental model reduces the direct responsibility of the healthcare services for illness by recognising the importance of environmental factors. But it also lays the services open to the claim that methods of diagnosis and treatment do not take enough account of the impact of poverty, stress and other aspects of people's lives on their state of health.

Looked at in terms of these models, healthcare successes are generally claimed by individuals and failures (even of individuals) are blamed on the service.

Language of the free market

The move towards a market economy is often seen in the media to have resulted in cutbacks and uneven distribution of provision. Media stories cite vastly different waiting times for the same treatments and tell of people travelling long distances to get care more quickly. The language of reporting has quickly adapted to take account of structural changes in how health care is funded and organised. Because the NHS itself speaks in the language of the marketplace, reporters echo the language back. So when Jaymee Bowen was refused treatment for leukaemia by Cambridgeshire Health Authority, the general perception was that the authority was not willing to 'waste' money on a child with a poor chance of survival. The media outcry deplored the state of the market-driven NHS which put cost-cutting before a child's life even though the health authority and professionals concerned insisted that it had been a decision based on clinical judgements and not on finance.

Victor and Penman (1995) analysed the problematic nature of language in the NHS and how this affects the way in which the health service is perceived by the public. The use of terms such as 'resource' gives people the idea that cost is now the dominant factor in planning healthcare provision, whether or not this is actually the case.

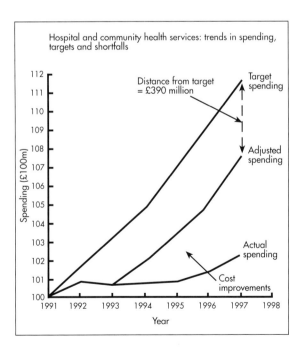

The graph alongside shows how the gap between the amount of money made available by the government and the amount healthcare researchers say is needed to maintain levels of service is widening. It shows:

- Actual spending — the amount made available by the government
- Adjusted spending — the amount made available by the government plus cost savings through improvements
- Target spending — the amount needed, based on the government's own estimate of resources required to fund the demands of an ageing population, modern technology and service improvements.

'Conservative Central Office is concerned that [*Casualty*] emphasises health cuts, under-staffing and low pay of the workforce.'
'BBC faces new Tory broadside'. *Observer*, November 2, 1986.

Images of healthcare professionals

Traditionally, healthcare professionals in the media are predominantly doctors and nurses. Until recently, there were few images of health visitors, midwives, paramedics, therapists, radiographers or counsellors.

Nursing stereotypes

Media images of nurses sometimes emphasise personality traits at the expense of skill and intellectual capacity. A DHSS survey (Rogers, 1984) found that nursing lacked credibility as a career among fifth and sixth formers, being seen as: 'not really relevant as a career for people with high intelligence because it involved humble jobs and offered little academic satisfaction'.

Four dominant nursing stereotypes (Bridges, 1990) are:

- *Ministering angel* — a nurturing, caring, selfless woman dedicated to her patients' care. This may appear at first an appealing or flattering image, at least to non-nurses. But it denies the nurse's personal identity, ambition, other areas of her experience and expertise. It also excludes men, as do all the stereotypes
- *Battle-axe* — may have originated in the power that Victorian matrons had over the personal and moral welfare of junior nurses. Stories of sadistic nurses seem to play on a deep-seated fear of vulnerability; a feminist view interprets this stereotype as a way of ridiculing the nurse at a time when the male patient is made vulnerable by illness
- *Naughty nurse* — the nurse as a flirtatious, sexually available woman. It is perhaps another response to the threatened potency of the man as patient, shifting responsibility for the sexually loaded situation of the man in bed in the woman's power onto the nurse: his vulnerability becomes a consequence of her blatant sexuality
- *Doctor's handmaiden* — someone with little independent spirit, experience, skill or decision-making capacity. She does the doctor's bidding and facilitates his care-giving and skill.

Stereotypes matter. They may undermine the confidence and self-esteem of nurses, affect the way patients view and interact with nurses and distort how policy-makers see nurses and allocate resources. They are also hard to overturn: a campaign in the mid-1980s which aimed to challenge myths and misconceptions about nursing suggested that the main task would be to break down the images of nursing and nurses routinely conveyed in the media (*Nursing Times*, 1983). TV

'Recent concern about the public image of the nurse...is not, at least directly, a product of feminist thought. Indeed it is remarkable to note how untouched British nurses and nursing are today by the feminist movement over the past two decades. In the United States, the almost obsessional interest in the profession's image is very much part of feminist preoccupations.'

Dunn, A. (1985/6) Images of nursing in the nursing and popular press. *Bulletin 9*, Winter 1985/6, of the History of Nursing Group at the Royal College of Nursing, pp2-8. London: RCN.

'To tackle the full force of a media which loves its nursing stereotypes — battleaxe, angel or whore — nursing must be very sure of its own ground... The next stage is to confront in a systematic way the images and stereotypes of nursing portrayed in the media. Already...nurses have shown us how to organise local groups to monitor press, TV and radio to ensure that whenever the wrong image of nursing is put forward, the presentation is challenged.

Nursing Times (Editorial). *Nursing Times* (1983) 79 (8): 21.

'Nurses as dedicated, selfless and angelic creatures, are good copy. Nurses in protest on picket lines create an image that runs counter to many of the clichés the downmarket papers have been gushing forth for some years.'

Vousden, M. (1988) What the papers said. *Nursing Times* 84 (7): 18.

programmes such as *Casualty* and *Cardiac Arrest* may have helped to overturn them, by showing doctors and healthcare professionals as a team. But it is important for nurses and other healthcare professionals to carry on working with the media to try to eradicate the stereotypes, particularly from tabloid newspaper coverage so that 'there is a continuity of interest between the profession and its patients' (Naish, 1990).

Yet perhaps the stereotypes have persisted in part because it has sometimes been in nurses' and doctors' interests to perpetuate them and in part because of the profession itself. As one commentator remarked at the start of the 1983 campaign: 'Is it just their image they want to change, as they claim? Or are they really seeking ways to change the profession itself?' (Toynbee, 1983). The debate about the profession has intensified since then, but all along it has been closely linked to the image of nursing. If doctors resist the rise in professional power and expertise of nurses, these stereotypes are a good way of keeping nurses 'in their place'. Further, 'these notions persist because nurses have not done enough to counteract them outside their own spheres, their own publications' (Dunn, 1985/6).

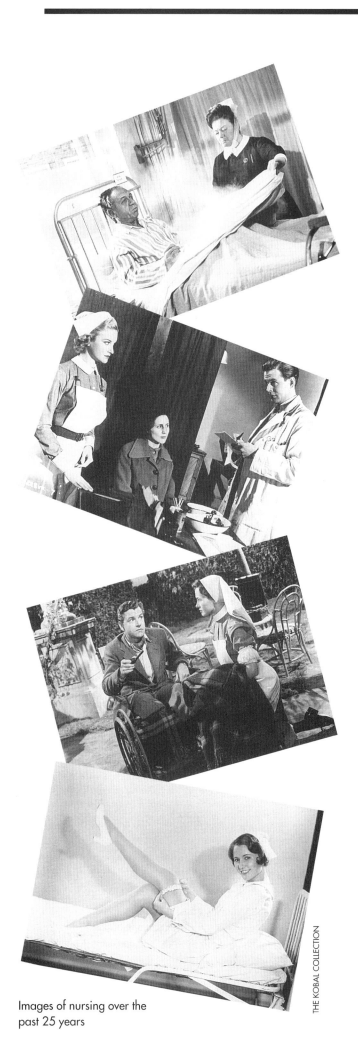

Images of nursing over the past 25 years

Conclusion

This Section looked at how people use the media and the different forms in which the media may present information about, or images of, health and health care.

The media have a pervasive influence on how people see, seek and use health care, on how they live and how they respond to illness. They bring important topics to public knowledge, uncover scandals and abuses and provide valuable information and advice. There are also negative impacts: scares can lead to panic which may be out of proportion to the threat; exposure of some issues at the expense of others can affect the allocation of funding and other resources — perhaps inappropriately in relation to the prevalence or severity of a problem. Furthermore, media coverage can be misleading, incomplete or even just wrong. This can lead to social effects such as stigmatisation of some groups, confusion over what constitutes healthy or suitable behaviour, or panic. However, public activity or opinion directed against established practices in health care (or any other area) need not be seen as inevitably negative. It may be a motivation for review, evaluation and change.

The role of the media in promoting healthy living, as in giving people accurate information, raises issues such as accountability and the moral or ethical functions of the media. It is not possible to look at only one area in isolation: influences on the media, the content of the media and the effects the media have are thoroughly intertwined.

'If it turns out that some families are able to benefit from publicity because they know how to manipulate the media, while others don't, then there is a whole new range of issues at the interface between journalism, medicine, and ethics.'

Karpf, A. (1988) *Doctoring the Media. The reporting of health and medicine*. London: Routledge.

What are these 'issues at the interface between journalism, medicine, and ethics'?

References

Bridges, J.M. (1990) Literature review on the images of the nurse and nursing in the media. *Journal of Advanced Nursing* 15(7): 850–854.

Cooper, G. (1995) Women sue top hospital over Down's test blunder. *Independent*, November 7, 1995.

Dixon, B. (1994) A rampant non-epidemic. *British Medical Journal* 308: 1576–1577.

Dunn, A. (1985/6) Images of nursing in the nursing and popular press. *Bulletin 9*, Winter 1985/6, of the History of Nursing Group at the Royal College of Nursing, pp2–8. London: RCN.

Eco, U. (1980) Towards a semiotic inquiry into the TV message. In: Corner, J. and Hawthorn, J. (eds) *Communication Studies: An introductory reader*. London: Arnold (4th edition, 1993).

Judge, K., Solomon, M., Miller, D. et al. (1992) Public opinion, the NHS and the media: changing patterns and perspectives. *British Medical Journal* 304: 893.

Karpf, A. (1988) *Doctoring the Media. The reporting of health and medicine*. London: Routledge.

McQuail, D. (1987) *Mass Communication Theory*. London: Sage Publications.

Miller, D. Kitzinger, J., Williams, K. et al (1992). Message misunderstood. *Times Higher Education Supplement*, July 3, 1992.

Morley, D. (1980) The *'Nationwide' Audience*. London: British Film Institute.

Naish, J. (1990) Hard-pressed angels. *Nursing Standard* 4(42): 17.

Neuberger, J. (1994) What sort of information should be available to the public in an open society? In: Marinker, M. (ed.) *Controversies in Health Care Policies: Challenges to practice*. London: British Medical Association.

Nursing Times (1983) Editorial. *Nursing Times* 79 (8): 21.

Otten, A.L. (1992) The influence of the mass media on health policy. *Health Affairs* Winter 1992: 111–118.

Platt, S. (1987) The aftermath of Angie's overdose: Is (soap) opera damaging to your health? *British Medical Journal* 294: 954–57.

Richardson, K. and Corner, J. (1986) Reading reception: Mediation and transparency in viewers' accounts of a TV programme. *Media, Culture and Society* 8(4): 485–508.

Rogers, R. (1984) The image makers. *Senior Nurse* 1(6): 10–11.

Smith, F. (1983) *Essays in Literacy*. London: Heinemann.

Toynbee, P. (1983) The ladies no longer have lamps. *World Medicine* 18 (11): 32.

Victor, P. and Penman, D. (1995) New NHS-speak has no word for compassion. *Independent on Sunday*, March 12, 1995.

Wober, J. (1987) *Informing the Public about AIDS*. London: Independent Broadcasting Authority.

Introduction

Most healthcare professionals do not have an insider's knowledge of the media unless they work with them as part of their job — someone who works in health promotion, for example, may have a closer view than a colleague working in clinical practice who sees the media from the outside. This book mainly takes the outside view, looking in. In this Section, you will be looking at the media the other way round, from the inside out. You will be seeing yourself, in your professional role and perhaps more generally as well, as a media person.

To help make the mental shift, ask yourself: 'What do I as a healthcare professional look like from the outsider's point of view of a patient or client?' You probably appear in at least three ways:

- As someone you might recognise — a human being to whom patients/clients relate in certain reasonably well defined and limited ways
- As a representative figure of 'hospital', 'medicine', 'ill health' — someone powerful, to be respected, perhaps feared and (in rare cases) an object of aggression and violence
- In the light of countless representations of nurses, doctors, midwives and so on, in the media and in conversations — you are part of a contemporary myth.

Media people probably appear in similar ways from the outside. The media are also to be respected, feared and sometimes hated. Media people are demonised, and sometimes lionised as well. They are also part of a contemporary myth.

Patients and clients may see healthcare professionals with the same eyes that you and they see the media. You are, for them, at least partly a media creation. What do these veils of miscomprehension and part-sense means, for you and them? How much do they matter? A starting point for this investigation is to recognise that from the perspective of the patient/client, every healthcare professional is part of the media. You are in the media room, the well-lit studio: learn to be comfortable there and to use its tricks.

'The glimpse of the interior through the doorway was more charming and mysterious than ever . . . It's the inside seen from the outside . . . that always seems so mysterious and wonderful.' Le Guin, U. (1995) In and out. In: *Searoad*. London: HarperCollins.

Watch two or three TV programmes which have media professionals being interviewed or taking part in a discussion. Before you watch, make up score sheets to record how well you think the participants do in the following areas:

- Appearing confident and relaxed, using appropriate body language that did not distract you
- Speaking clearly and concisely with authority
- Taking the lead sometimes rather than letting the other participants dominate.

There may be other factors you want to record. Watching and analysing how the professionals perform will help you understand what lies 'through the doorway'.

Presenting . . . what?

The traditional positive picture of healthcare professionals is of people who are dedicated to their patients/clients and committed to the ethos of public service. This is a powerful image, which is powerfully amplified in the media, and it brings a fund of goodwill from the public. Healthcare professionals live with the image because they see the TV programmes and read the papers like everyone else: they also live it, consciously or not. Every time they put on a uniform to go on a ward, they also put on the mantle of their profession in a figurative sense. This applies as much to healthcare professionals who do not wear a uniform. It's not the clothes that count, it's the image.

The upside

What is the image made up of? Mostly it is the attributes of a role rather than the personal attributes of a particular personality. Work roles can give people great strength and authority (though they can also take them away). Individual healthcare professionals can draw strength from the shared understanding of their broad role as carers: there is a consensus in society that they are there to do good.

As well as this very broad current of approval from society, healthcare professionals also draw strength from being part of:

- *A profession* — with its own professional values and standards and a long history of public service
- *An organisation* — a hospital or community trust, with its physical and psychological presence in an area and its concentration of expertise
- *A team* — with colleagues who think and act in similar ways, pursuing a common end of patient/client care.

All this provides a highly supportive setting for the individual.

The downside

Of course, there is a downside as well which puts the positive image constantly under siege. If there is a fear that the National Health Service is being run down and privatised, people who work in it become victims as well as heroines.

Healthcare professionals are very conscious of this other side of reality, the dark side. They live it just as much as they live the positive side. They experience directly the effect of cuts, staff

'There is no such thing as society. There are individuals, and there are families.'
Margaret Thatcher, quoted in: Young, H. (1989). *One of Us. A biography of Margaret Thatcher*. London: Macmillan.

'When you have people saying there is no such thing as society, it is rather like finding yourself back in the 17th century with people saying that the earth is flat.'
Peter Townsend, quoted in: Richards, H. (1996) Warrior on want. *Times Higher Education Supplement* August 30, 1996.

Trusts and health authorities may be wary about healthcare professionals talking to the press. They worry that employees will say something critical or unguarded and they have come to associate media coverage with bad press.

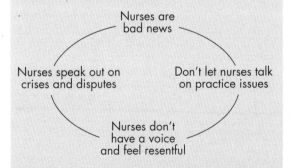

Nurses appear in the media when there are problems — pay disputes, complaints about shortages and cut-backs. The assumption is that a nurse on the news is bad for the corporate image, and to prevent nurses talking to the press on other issues, so perpetuating the myth.

shortages and budget ceilings and see the impact on patient/client care. Sometimes, inevitably, this dark image gets played out in the way they present themselves to their patients or clients — harassed, overworked, exhausted and perhaps short-tempered. Healthcare professionals, like everyone else, do not perform best under this sort of stress. Such an image also gets played out in the media, which weaves another thread into the never-ending story: hospitals are full of managers who follow the dictates of commerce not care, doctors who are asleep on their feet, shut wards and empty beds, poor quality equipment...and so on. It's all good copy; grist to the media mill.

Mixed messages

The mixed messages presented by healthcare professionals, in their real selves and their media 'doubles', reflect the reality of their working lives. Mixed messages can also be seen in the way that trusts present themselves through their own media:

- Glossy brochures; full-colour illustrated magazines for board members; newsletters for staff; smart press conferences to launch new initiatives — an image of high quality, the public face saying: 'This is what we are like'

- Tatty notices in staff rooms and in wards; low-budget leaflets for health promotion — an image not necessarily of low quality but of the daily reality of tight budgets and not enough time to concentrate on anything but the essentials of patient/client care.

Are nurses and other healthcare professionals more likely than doctors to be 'bad news' for trust and health authority managers, in your view? What difference is being made to this defensive attitude by the growing willingness of doctors to speak out against the consequences of cuts in the health services?

You might like to trace the mixed messages that doctors and healthcare professionals give in the media as part of your assessment for this unit. You could produce a matrix showing the extent to which they express:

- Support for their organisation and criticism of the government
- Criticism of both organisation and government
- Support for both.

Newsletters such as *Target*, published by the Department of Health to disseminate *Health of the Nation* initiatives, help to strengthen feelings of worth and solidarity in the profession. As well as articles describing projects they contain morale-boosting messages such as this one from the chief medical officer, Sir Kenneth Calman:

'What we're seeing is health beginning to change. That's not from the top. It's from the bottom and that's the exciting thing.'

Target, Issue 6, May 16, 1996.

Presenting well

What lies behind the self-assured, effective presentation of a media professional, a politician who comes over well on the TV and radio or a trust spokesperson who appears to be articulate and authoritative? These two pages look at how presentation skills help to get across a message. These skills are generic; they are not reserved for media professionals. They are as useful for presenting effectively to colleagues in multi-professional teams or to members of the public, including patients and clients, as they are to those at a press conference. People use the skills of presentation on one another all the time.

Know what you are doing

'A presenter is much closer to an advocate than to a teacher or lecturer. A presentation is an exercise in persuasion' (Jay, 1972). Media professionals tailor their message to their audience. Jay identifies three dimensions of this. His advice is meant for formal presentations lasting 30 or 40 minutes, such as at a conference, but it also holds good when presenting informally, for much shorter periods:

- *Texture* — vary the means of communication, including solid talk, visuals and ad lib. remarks
- *Attention curve* — take account of variations in the level of attention, high in the first 10 minutes, dropping more and more steeply in the next 20 minutes or so and lifting five minutes before the end
- *Impact* — keep the audience alert and alive to the main points.

It is also important to pitch the level of knowledge and complexity of discourse at the right level. For example, if a doctor or healthcare professional is being interviewed or writing an article for a professional journal, they can assume that the readers will have a good grounding in medical practice, and possibly the appropriate area of health care. They assume some common knowledge, an understanding of technical terms and some of the background to the issue. On the other hand, if they are on a radio phone-in answering questions about a local meningitis outbreak, the approach will be different. They will need to give :

- A clear, simple explanation of the risks
- Information on what to look out for
- Information on what to do in suspected cases.

Watch a newscaster or other professional TV communicator. Look at the person's body language, posture and the content and style of the presentation. How is the person making the communication accessible?

How do these communicators overcome the barrier of media being largely a one-way channel?

An Eastern proverb goes: 'I hear and forget, I see and remember, I do and understand'. Next time you go to a conference or a presentation by a colleague or manager, notice to what extent and how successfully they:

- Get across their message in words alone
- Use visual images to make points and keep the audience's attention
- Get the audience participating.

Here are some guidelines for presenters:

- Avoid irritating mannerisms, but use normal body language
- Make sure your jewellery, or change in your pocket, doesn't jangle as you move
- Smile when appropriate — but not too much
- Make eye contact with people in the audience — not always the same person
- Don't look directly into a TV camera unless told to; look at the interviewer
- Respond to other people to show you are taking notice — it makes the communication as two-way as possible
- Let your hands hang at your sides while standing — don't clench your fists or put your hands in your pockets.

Structure of presentations

Mandel (1987) suggests that 'All effective presentations make the pattern of organisation crystal clear to the audience'. He proposes a hierarchy of:

* *Main ideas* — these could include general assertions such as 'We need to review the way clinical supervision is working'
* *Sub-ideas* — including explanations, data, evidence and other specifics to support the main ideas
* *Introduction and conclusion.*

Good presenters give 'markers' to help the audience identify the most important parts of the message. They put the main points first, or outline them before launching into details. This gives people clues as to the content and structure of the presentation, and if anyone gives up before the end they will still have had a brief summary of the most important points. Again, the advice is good for less formal presentations, such as explaining case notes to colleagues.

One-way communication

The communication skills used in everyday interactions with others are essentially two-way. We judge people's response to our messages from:

* Questions they ask; interruptions
* Their expression, posture and body language
* Tone of voice and the type of language they use when replying
* Non-verbal sounds such as 'ums', which may be encouraging or dismissive.

When talking to the media, viewers, listeners or readers cannot interact or give their responses. Good media presenters talk 'through' the reporter to the people they are really addressing; as the radio journalist Sue MacGregor says: 'Always imagine there are a lot of people out there who really do want to hear what you have to say' (MacGregor, 1992). If you want to see how it's done, watch a television interview with a skilled politician.

A current view in health promotion is that healthcare professionals should demonstrate positive personal qualities rather than any particular sort of behaviour or presentation. The sorts of personal qualities that are important include:

* Having knowledge
* Knowing the choices
* Being able to create new choices or options
* Making decisions
* Making choices using their own definition of health.

Personal qualities such as genuineness, warmth, empathy and trust, which make intimacy possible, are at least as important as good health-related behaviours. The challenge for healthcare professionals is to:

* Discover positive aspects of themselves which are appropriate to role models
* Feel good about these discoveries and legitimise or validate them in terms of prevalent thinking about the nature of health.

Clarke, A. (1991) Nurses as role models and health educators. *Journal of Advanced Nursing* 16: 1178-84.

Read the guidelines for presenters on the page opposite. Isn't it just common sense, ordinary behaviour? Why do people need this advice just because they are presenting something? Wouldn't you feel and do better presenting yourself in the way you normally would?

There is more on effective communication with individuals and groups, including the importance of body language and tones of voice, in the unit *Professional Relationships: Influences on health care.*

Taking part

Occasionally, healthcare professionals may find themselves on a radio or TV programme, or being interviewed for a newspaper or magazine. More often, they may contribute to a newsletter or professional journal with an article or letter. As with presentations (see pages 108-109), the skills used when engaging with the media in these ways are transferable to other contexts. If healthcare professional think of themselves as media people in their communications with patients, clients and colleagues, then all the skills of a good media communicator come into play, including:

- *Careful listening* — to understand the issue being discussed, or hear what the question is
- *Sensitivity* — to what the other people are thinking and to any hidden messages
- *Preparation* — so as not to be taken by surprise or left without an answer
- *Tact and diplomacy* — knowing how to word an answer indirectly, or how to side-step questions that are inappropriate or too difficult to answer at the time.

Preparation

If healthcare professionals are approached by someone in the media, or through the PR department of a trust or health authority, to communicate on an issue via some aspect of the media, getting answers to questions such as the following will help to determine the type of contribution they are expected to make:

- Is it a documentary feature or a news item?
- Will they appear with others or alone?
- How much time will they be given?

To prepare in advance for media-type contacts, it is advisable to:

- Think about the points you want to make and how you are going to make them
- Observe any limitations on what you can say, whether these are legal constraints or ethical restrictions
- Be aware of how what you say may be used and how it may be misinterpreted.

It is normally good to come across as competent and confident both in professional practice and on the media. This may mean knowing the facts — such as how long people have to wait for routine surgery; or being clear about an opinion — for example, the reasons for supporting a call

There are some formalities that people observe when they are in the spotlight, to help them come across well and provide protection from saying wrong or inappropriate things. For example, healthcare professionals need to bear in mind:

- *Patients' rights* — not discussing individual cases in a way that would enable patients to be identified

- *Clauses in their contracts limiting access to the media* — it's worth checking with the authority or PR department

- *The law on libel and slander* — this protects individuals and organisations from unfair accusations.

Media reports can have an element of sleight of hand:

'I was surprised at how deceptive it all was. I was taped in an interview with a single reporter, and then it was mixed with interviews from other people and presented as though it were a round table discussion, even though we'd never met and certainly weren't responding to other people's comments.'

Christine, interviewed by BBC Radio.

'I recorded my contribution in Cambridge, though the other people taking part in the discussion were in London. I could hear them and knew the format of the programme, but it wouldn't be obvious to viewers that I was in a different studio.'

Bill, interviewed by BBC Radio.

for industrial action. If there are likely to be questions which need statistics or other evidence, it may help to get them in advance so you can hand them out, particularly if you are talking to the press. If you think you will be asked for an opinion about anything, it is good to know roughly what you want to say, but don't script it or you won't sound natural.

'Voice'

People often come across well on the broadcast media, whether they are professional broadcasters, politicians who are used to it or ordinary people, because their voice sounds right. This is more a matter of being natural, relaxed and confident than the actual, physical business of voice production. There is a link, however, between feeling relaxed and sounding (or looking) it. The quality of someone's 'voice' is also partly a result of the quality of their ideas and the way they are articulated. It includes a sense of humour, lack of dogmatism, willingness to listen and the ability to think quickly and come up with an appropriate response.

Control

Reporters and interviewers often like to take control. This is partly because they are responsible for the quality of the programme or article. If they sense that someone is confident, articulate and has something interesting to say, they are more likely to relax the controls. The same holds good in other contexts and it can lead to much better communication. For example, in a formal meeting or job interview, a confident and articulate participant can usually create the 'space' to talk about his or her ideas and give an impression of their personality. Such people come across well, just as some people do on the TV or radio.

With two colleagues or others in your tutor/counsellor group, agree an issue on which you could be interviewed. It may be some topical national issue, or something specific to your work setting.

One of you works out some questions to ask. The second person responds to the questions. The third watches and notes down:

What sorts of questions they were — for example, friendly, hostile, tricky, straightforward.

How the person being interviewed responded — confidently, unconfidently, with a straight answer, diplomatically.

Afterwards, review how it went. What lessons can be learned about taking part in these sorts of situations?

'Be yourself — don't try and sound like someone else or someone you would like to be. But be your 'best' self, the confident one, the one that responds well to other people. Don't forget that you are with two sets of people: the interviewer or others on the programme if it's a panel and the audience. If the interviewer or other people on the programme are hostile, you don't have to respond to them with hostility. You tend to come across as defensive or rude if you do that. Talk to the audience instead, because you'll probably feel better about them. And don't be afraid of your own ideas and ways of saying things.'

Local politician

'Soundbite: a brief segment on television news in which a reporter, or political figure, etc. delivers a short succinct report or statement.'

Chambers Dictionary (1994) Edinburgh: Chambers Harrap Publishers Ltd.

Politics and the profession

It can be difficult to combine a professional status and union membership, particularly in a political climate where unions are seen in oppositional terms. One of the consequences of political and media attacks on unions over the past 15 years is that the unions themselves — and their members — sometimes come across as defensive. How do healthcare professionals feel about the ways in which these issues are portrayed in the media? As media activists themselves, how do they present their involvement in issues of pay, contracts and conditions of service to others, including patients/clients and other colleagues?

In the news

News coverage of professionals such as doctors, solicitors or university lecturers usually focuses on their expertise, or occasionally their mistakes. News about healthcare workers tends to focus less on what they do and more on how well (or badly) they are paid, what happens or might happen when they take industrial action and how they negotiate working conditions.

Since 1979, the government has been unwilling to become directly involved in sorting out industrial disputes. As management and workers in the public service sector fight it out on their own, disputes have moved into the public eye and in front of the television camera. In the past decade, industrial disputes have been increasingly fought out in the media, particularly the broadcast media, rather than around the negotiating table. Instead of a private meeting, televised statements from opposing factions or a televised dispute have become the normal mode of progress. There is often a close and co-operative relationship between the management and union leaders in a dispute: both are working towards a resolution and both recognise the importance of the media.

Nurses' day of action, February 3, 1988

Nurses are in an unusual position when they take industrial action because they start with a large bank of public goodwill and sympathy. Even so, news coverage of the nurses' day of action in 1988 was not wholly sympathetic. On the day of the action, the *Sun* printed an article sympathising with the financial plight of the nurses. The next day, it applauded the nurses who did work and minimised the impact of the call to strike; it also blamed 'red yobbos' for hijacking the day of action. The *Guardian* supported the striking nurses. Its coverage on the

---

The Daily Telegraph: 'Hospital strike backed by only 2%.'

Guardian: 'Thousands protest.'

'Of course, '2% of nurses' and 'thousands' are the same thing but the word 'only' is editorial comment itself.'

Vousden, M. (1988) What the papers said. *Nursing Times* 84: 7, 18.

Junior doctors' hours have received a lot of media attention. How has this issue about hours — or a similar issue concerning medical staff — been covered? Is it seen predominantly as an area of professional practice or as industrial dispute? What are the issues raised by the debate? Would the same issues be raised for nurses and other healthcare professionals?

What incompatibilities do you feel in your role as a professional and a union member?

To what extent are you aware of displaying a different 'image' from your normal professional persona when you are talking about issues of pay, conditions and service, or strike action?

How does this affect the way you talk to people about these issues?

The National Union of Journalists has a code of professional conduct that lays out the basis of good journalistic practice.

day after concentrated on how responsible strikers had been in making sure emergency cover was available, on the carnival atmosphere at some hospitals and clinics and on the obstinacy and perceived incompetence of the government.

The nurses' strike proved difficult to assimilate into the established framework for representations of nurses. Some parts of the media found it so difficult to reconcile their image of 'angels' with industrial action that they resorted to blaming other influences. Coverage 'exposed the dilemma many papers faced in reconciling the idea of angelic nurses on the picket line. Many solved this by suggesting that nurses were somehow being led astray by left wing agitators' (Vousden, 1988). So the *Sun* ran headlines such as 'Nurse arrested as red wreckers hijack demo' (February 4, 1988). The body copy was no better: 'Militant left wing troublemakers muscled in on the nurses' first ever national strike yesterday —bringing fury and violence to a peaceful protest...the jeering rent-a-mob lefties pushed uniformed nurses into a police cordon of officers with linked arms'. The nurses' responsibility for their choice was denied and their cause subsumed in an attack on the left.

The ambulance drivers' strike

How industrial disputes are covered in the media affects people's perception of the group taking action. Sophisticated public relations (PR) techniques are used to direct or manipulate media coverage. The ambulance drivers' strike of 1989 was one health workers' dispute where PR machinery was used to the full (see pages 114-115 for more on PR). The ambulance drivers needed public sympathy and support for their case. They made it publicly known that some were working without pay to maintain a skeleton service to give the public some level of protection. The message was clear — they were against the government but for the public. The ambulance drivers also found incidents to report on a regular basis to keep the dispute in the public eye: the *Times* index lists 115 items on the dispute published in the *Times* between June 1, and December 31, 1989.

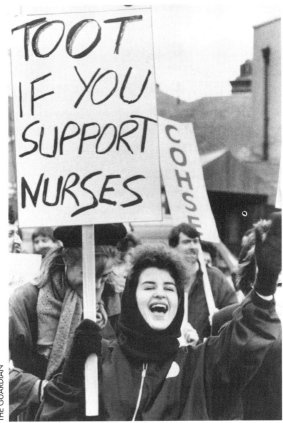

THE GUARDIAN

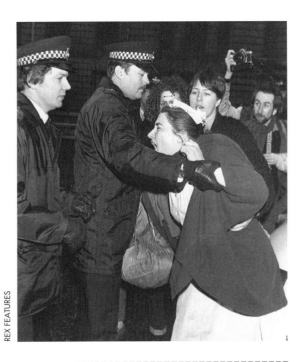

REX FEATURES

Why did the *Sun* and the *Guardian* choose these images to illustrate their stories of striking nurses? How do you react to them? Try them out on your patients/clients to see how they react.

Public relations

In a sense, anyone who has anything to do with the public in a professional capacity is part of public relations (PR). Arguably, the most important form of public relations for a trust or health authority is made up of things that healthcare professionals do and the way they come across to patients, clients, funding body representatives and other stakeholders in the health service. Every time you relate to someone outside your immediate team, you are part of PR.

Some people are employed as PR professionals. Their role is to manage the interface between their organisation or client and the media. They:
- Catch the attention of people who make the news
- Open channels of communication between an organisation and the media, for example by finding people for media representatives to interview
- Manage external relations and the image conveyed in public announcements.

The public relations business has grown rapidly over the past decade. Many organisations now have a PR department or press office which issues statements, plans publicity events and

may also handle advertising. Individuals may use a PR consultant if they have extensive dealings with the media or a high profile role in society. Trade unions, pressure groups, charities, actors, hospital and community trusts and members of the royal family now have PR advisers.

The growth of the PR function means that people are less likely to talk to the press in an unguarded or untutored way. In organisations with a PR department, employees are usually expected to consult the department before making any public statement or appearance. Statements are carefully worded, speakers groomed and events orchestrated to create the most beneficial effects and impressions.

Press releases and conferences

One of the important functions of a PR department is to write press releases and field inquiries from the press. It may also occasionally organise press conferences, launches and other events to which media representatives are invited. A press release is a written statement sent to selected media organisations. It is carefully worded and may be embargoed until a certain date. This means that although the media have access to the information, they are

Arrange a visit to the PR department of your trust or health authority. Ask when you plan your visit if you can interview the manager or another member of the staff. Use the interview to find out exactly what they do. They may be able to show you the media coverage that resulted from one of their activities.

Reflect on what you found out. You could ask yourself functional questions such as:

- What function does the PR department fulfil?

- Should health service resources be used in this way?

- How could you or colleagues you work with make use of the PR facilities?

Or you could ask questions that relate to your role in public relations, for example:

What PR techniques can I use or adapt in my own work?

What do these techniques teach me about how to relate to other people in a professional way?

not allowed to publish or broadcast it until a specified time. There is an established tradition of respecting embargoes, though they are occasionally breached. The embargo procedure enables papers and magazines to prepare copy in advance so that the news can be reported immediately on the release date.

Press releases are written carefully to catch the eye of the news editor and make it attractive as it stands. If it suits the style of a magazine or newspaper, a press release may be used with few changes, so it is usually specially tailored to the publications it is sent to. Local newspapers, which are run to tight budgets, are more likely than national papers to reproduce a press release undigested.

A press (or news) conference is a meeting between the media and representatives of an organisation, or an individual. It is called for a reason, for example to announce new developments, report on progress, or respond to criticism or earlier press coverage. At a press conference, one or more people will make a statement to the press. This will have been carefully worded and written or vetted by a PR department or professional. The speakers may

accept questions from the media representatives present. There will probably be a photo call — an opportunity for press photographers to take photographs of the people (and possibly objects) central to the press conference. In some cases, a press conference is only a statement with no opportunity for questions. It is then much the same in effect as a press release.

When an organisation sends out a press release or arranges a photo opportunity, it likes to feel in control of the images and text which will be used. But sometimes the media undercut the official line and make a different statement from that originally intended. It is easy to subvert the official message and convey a subtext that is critical of it or refutes it.

Sometimes PR goes badly wrong. In 1990, agriculture minister John Gummer agreed to a photo opportunity to demonstrate the safety of beef by showing his family eating it. One of the invited photographers stood away from the others (you can see the rest in the background of the picture) and took a photo of the minister apparently force-feeding his reluctant four-year-old daughter Cordelia with a hamburger. The photo became the enduring record of the staged event. It was used on the cover of the following week's *Private Eye*, and the *Guardian* awarded Gummer first prize for the most counter-productive image of 1990.

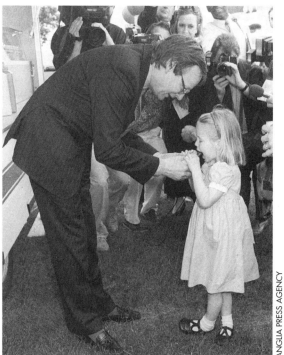

'The gruesome spectacle of the agriculture minister and his daughter cramming their mouths with what the nation instantly christened BSE-burgers.'
Caulkin, S. (1990) Mad cows and a pig's ear.
Guardian, July 16, 1990

Presenting information

A press release is an example of how to exercise control over information. Unlike an interview, the person writing a press release is in charge of the questions that get answered and the amount of information provided. Press releases are pieces of writing that follow certain rules. The rules hold good for a lot of writing and may apply just as well to other forms of communication where it is important to control the flow of information — for example, if some of the information is confidential or if it is complex. Writing within the rules is often a good way of getting something complicated straightened out.

Public relations professionals use press releases so that they can communicate with the media on their own terms. The sender controls what is sent out and can spend time preparing the material to present exactly the message and image wanted. Once it is out of the sender's hands, what the media do with the information will depend on:

- How good the press release is — if it is well written, they may use chunks of it as it stands
- How much space/time they have to cover the story
- Their agenda — there is not much that the PR professional can do to alter this.

The rules of writing

A press release works well if it tells a good story. The same is true of a lot of writing:

- Write in a punchy, straightforward style without jargon
- Make the main points clear
- Structure the text so that the most interesting items come first, and amplification of them follows
- Include case history or personal interest material if appropriate
- Do not include irrelevant information or any information you do not want to get out
- Give contact details so that people can get hold of you for further information or other resources, such as illustrations.

Information is usually best presented in a fairly simple format. Press releases and similar forms of communication do not have to look as polished as a finished article, although they may contain text that can be used directly in an article. The less work there is to do with a press release, the more likely it is to be used by a news department pressed for time. The same might be true of a piece of news for an internal newsletter at work:

- Do not use fancy text styles and complicated layouts

'In conjunction with tissue samples taken as part of this study, definitive information should become available as to whether SIDS deaths were associated in any way with the use of fire-retardant chemicals. Results of the expanded CESDI studies will not be available for analysis until the autumn of 1996...Further data from the studies that we have set in train need to be available and assessed before we can produce a final report. At all stages of our deliberations we have asked the question: "Is there any evidence of risk to infants?" To date we have seen none.'

DoH press release. *1st interim report to chief medical officer from the expert group to investigate cot death theories.* London: DoH, December 8, 1995.

'Cot death fumes link disproved

'Scientists have found no evidence that mattresses contribute to cot deaths by producing deadly fumes...'

Guardian, December 8, 1995.

Look at the two extracts in the box alongside — one from a statement by an expert group and the other from an article written from it. Do you think the article fairly represents the parts of the statement you can see? How and why has the journalist changed the emphasis?

Here is a possible format for a press release:

Details of who sent the press release
Date
Topic of press release
Statistics and other relevant facts
Contact details for further information
Title
Body text

'Ends' or 'Continues' (to tell readers if there are more sheets they should have)
List any enclosures or attachments.

- Leave large margins and use double-spacing so that people can make notes on the page
- Print it clearly on one side of the paper only
- Refer to any attached or enclosed materials, such as photographs, so that if they get separated the reader knows to look for them.

Using pictures

Newspapers and magazines like 'visuals', that is, illustrations, photographs and charts — they liven up the page, help people to understand the story and can be interesting or entertaining in their own right. If you are writing for publication, include appropriate photographs or other types of illustrations. For black and white photographs, send large black and white prints. For colour photographs, send transparencies. These should preferably be large format, not the 35mm film that most cameras take. If you are having photographs taken professionally, you can ask for this format. For other illustrations, clear line drawings or charts and graphs produced on a computer and printed clearly on a laser printer are best.

'The original, commonest, easiest-to-produce kind of interaction is that between people. If you are stuck writing or trying to figure something out, there is nothing better than finding one person, or more, to talk to...Two heads are better than one because two heads can make conflicting material interact better than one head usually can.'

Elbow, P. (1973) *Writing Without Teachers*. Oxford: Oxford University Press.

Writing a press release may help you pick up certain rules that you can then transfer into other sorts of writing. Ask the PR department of your trust or health authority if you can see some of the press releases they have sent out recently. See if you can identify a common format and structure. Make up a template for yourself to help you write a press release in the same way.

Pick an event or report relating to your area of practice and write a press release about it. You may be able to ask someone in the PR office to comment on it for you, or you could discuss it with colleagues.

Advertising and editorial

Except for the BBC, all the media mix advertising with editorial content. Advertisements are one way of getting across a message. They have disadvantages from the point of view of their producers: they normally have to be paid for and there is a danger that the general perception of advertisements as 'always trying to sell you something' will dilute the message. For viewers, readers and listeners they are an integral part of the 'flow' of communication (see pages 52–53). Like other forms of content, they can be anywhere between the centre of attention and the periphery.

The function of advertising is to translate the world of things (objects) into a vocabulary of desire, creating connections and links that are symbols of exchange — and that lead to an actual exchange of money for goods or services. Judith Williamson (1994) has traced the process of increasing sophistication in the form of advertising over the past 20 years. She comments that advertisements now show a 'skilful, self-conscious use of semiotics', but that their basic intention is still the same: 'Advertisements *intend* to make us feel we are lacking'.

Advertising what?

Advertisements can be for:

- Products that are unhealthy, such as cigarettes and sweets
- Products that are good for us, such as fresh fruit
- Healthcare products and services, such as drugs and cosmetic surgery.

Advertising for things that are generally acknowledged as unhealthy either ignore the risk or play on it. The slogan 'naughty but nice', advertising cream cakes, played on people's guilt at eating something they know is bad for them but defused the guilt by making it flippant, almost a game. The choice of the word 'naughty' is associated with children and minor misdeeds and has a mild sexual connotation. It draws attention away from the serious health risk of a bad diet.

The occasional cream cake is not likely to be harmful for most people, so the 'naughty but nice' tactic can work. But it probably wouldn't work with cigarette advertising, because the threat is perceived as more serious. Advertising for cigarettes and alcohol plays down the risk — and the information content — by concentrating

'The ads are by far the best part of any magazine or newspaper. More pains and thought, more wit and art go into the making of an ad than into any prose feature of press or magazine. Ads are news. What is wrong with them is that they are always good news. In order to balance off the effect and to sell good news, it is necessary to have a lot of bad news.'
McLuhan, M. (1964) *Understanding Media: The extensions of man*. London: Routledge (reprinted 1994).

'...a diamond comes to "mean" love and endurance for us. Once the connection has been made, we begin to translate the other way and in fact to skip translating altogether: taking the sign for what it signifies, the thing for the feeling.'
Williamson, J. (1994) *Decoding Advertisements: Ideology and meaning in advertising*. London: Marion Boyars (4th impression).

'Publicity is the life of this culture — in so far as without publicity capitalism could not survive — and at the same time publicity is its dream.'
Berger, J. (1990) *Ways of Seeing*. Harmondsworth: Penguin Books.

Survey the mix of advertising and editorial in one general interest magazine and one professional journal. Compare the number of advertisements for different sorts of products and services: healthy, unhealthy, healthcare products. Some advertisements will not fall into any of these categories and you could invent your own. Look at how the advertisements work and to what extent they support the general editorial content of the publication or undermine it.

What is the degree of disjunction (see pages 90–91)?

What effect does this have on you as a reader?

This Activity could form part of your assessment for the unit, if you combine it with other Activities investigating the content of media publications.

British Rate and Data (BRAD) is a monthly publication that gives advertising rates for print and broadcast media. If you want to find out the cost of the advertisements you see in magazines, look at a copy in a library.

on cryptic or appealing visuals. The advertisement promises a sophisticated or macho lifestyle, or invites people to join the élite group of those who can decode the advertisement. A sense of belonging can produce a feeling of empathy with the product.

There is not nearly as much advertising for healthy products as for unhealthy ones. But healthy food is sometimes used in advertisements as a way of promoting a positive, healthy image. Supermarket advertisements show a lot of fresh fruit and vegetables, although most of their profit comes from selling convenience foods and household goods. Baby food manufacturers show piles of fresh ingredients they want people to believe are used in their product. Advertisements in the general press for remedies usually show a reassuring image, either of how nice life will be if you take them, or a more abstract picture that conveys a feeling of well-being associated with the remedy. Healthcare products advertised include:

- Self-help remedies, such as headache cures, cold remedies, pregnancy tests, toothpaste and vitamin supplements
- Private clinics, most of which are cosmetic surgery clinics

- Drugs and appliances available on prescription (in professional healthcare journals).

Does advertising fit the editorial?
The message of some advertisements is reinforced by the editorial. For example, diet supplements are advertised alongside editorial pages featuring ultra-thin models, and cosmetic surgery advertisements come between images of perfectly-proportioned women and advice on looking beautiful. Even if the editors would not advocate cosmetic surgery, an overall message of the magazine is usually that it is important to look conventionally attractive.

A special type of advertising is the health promotion messages sponsored by the Department of Health and other organisations. Health promotion differs from other advertising. It may try to persuade people not to do something they might want to do — don't smoke, don't drink too much, don't have sex without using a condom; it is not selling anything. But it is not always effective.

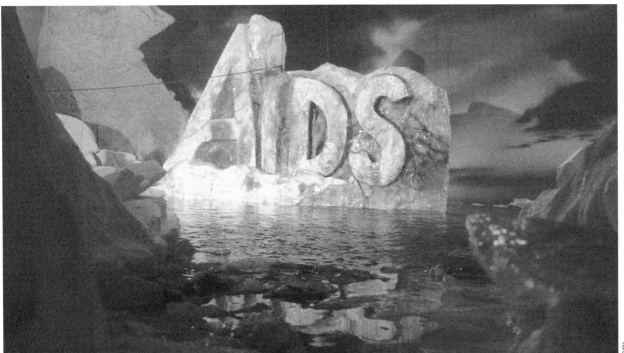

Why did the Aids campaign using the 'iceberg' not work?

There is more on how the media can be actively used to promote health in the unit *Health Promotion in Professional Practice*.

Conclusion

This Section has summarised some of the skills media people use in their work. There are many areas of professional practice in which media skills can benefit you directly, such as:

- Producing health promotion or information videos
- Producing leaflets, posters, information sheets
- Running a campaign and producing press releases for it.

There are also many areas where these skills form part of your ability and competence as a healthcare professional, such as:

- Listening and talking to patients, clients and colleagues
- Presenting a positive image of yourself, your team, organisation and profession
- Writing clearly and succinctly for different purposes.

Seeing yourself as a media person, someone who can make use of many of the skills that media professionals use, should help to professionalise these areas of your work. It should also give you an insight into the way patients/clients see you. As an active, canny participant in the media world — the world of today — you might also be developing a greater sense of control over the way you allow the media themselves to become implicated in your life. In a psychological sense, the aim might be to integrate the media so that you are able to act autonomously despite their constant presence and influence.

Overall, the material in this book should prove valuable in many areas of your practice, by enabling you to:

- Analyse and understand healthcare stories in the press and broadcast media, and anticipate some of the effects they may have on the public in general and on groups of patient/clients

- Understand how people's ideas about health and illness, the NHS and healthcare professionals are formed

- Identify bias, partiality or a particular angle in a story and work out the implications for how it will be received and how it will affect people

- Get your message across effectively when dealing with the media yourself

- Critically evaluate literature, videos and other materials you come across in your practice intended either to inform or educate practitioners or to help patients/clients

- Communicate more effectively with patients/clients and other healthcare professionals.

References

Jay, A. (1972) *Effective Presentation*. London: British Institute of Management.

MacGregor, S. (1992) Quoted in: *A Guide to Handling the Media: The television interview*. Bristol: BBS productions.

Mandel, S. (1987) *Effective Presentation Skills*. London: Kogan Page.

Vousden, M. (1988) What the papers said. *Nursing Times* 84(7): 18.

Williamson J. (1994) *Decoding Advertisements: Ideology and meaning in advertising*. London: Marion Boyars (4th impression).

Write an account in your learning journal of what you have learned practising some of the Activities described in this Section.

How do you view the media, now that you have tried out some of the production processes?

Do you think you would like to work more closely with the media? Are there ways in which you might extend your practice to give you a chance to do this? Some examples are:

- Becoming involved with your local community or hospital radio

- Offering to write on healthcare issues for a local newspaper, free sheet or community newsletter

- Suggesting a health-related programme idea to your local radio or television station

- Starting a newsletter for your area of practice

- Asking the PR department of your trust or health authority to bear you in mind if they are asked to find a practitioner to interview or to appear on a broadcast.

Think about what you could do, and make a few notes in your journal on your plans. If you carry them through, you might like to write an evaluation of your experience and how it matched your expectations. This might form part of your assessment for the unit.